中医药问答六百三十题

630
Questions & Answers
about
Chinese Herbal Medicine
A Workbook & Study Guide

by

Bob Flaws

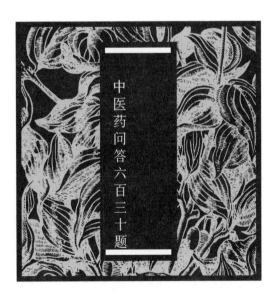

中医药问答六百三十题

BLUE • POPPY • PRESS

Published by:

Blue Poppy Press
A Division of Blue Poppy Enterprises, Inc.
3450 Penrose Place, Suite 110
Boulder, CO 80301
(303) 447-8372

First Edition February, 1999

ISBN 1-891845-04-7
Library of congress Catalog Card #98-94962

The information in this book is given in good faith. However, the author and the
publishers cannot be held responsible for any error or omission. Nor can
they be held in any way responsible for treatment given on the basis of information
contained in this book. The publishers make this information available to English
readers for scholarly and research purposes only.

The publishers do not advocate nor endorse self-medication by laypersons. Chinese
medicine is a professional medicine. Laypersons interested in availing themselves
of the treatments described in this book should seek out a
qualified professional practitioner of Chinese medicine.

COMP Designation: Connotative translation

Printed at Johnson Printing
Cover design by Anne Rue

10, 9, 8, 7, 6, 5, 4, 3, 2

Preface

This book is meant as an aid for the study of Chinese herbal medicine. It can also be used to help prepare for Chinese herbal examinations, be they school course exams or state and national licensing/certification exams. It contains over 630 sample questions on all aspects of Chinese herbal medicine. In general, one must have a good grasp of the following areas of expertise before one can be said to be knowledgeable in Chinese herbal medicine:

Materia medica:

Categorization
Natures (i.e., temperatures)
Flavors
Channel-enterings
Functions
Indications
Doses
Contraindications or prohibitions
Commonly used combinations
Methods of preparation & administration

Formulas:

Categorization
Ingredients
Functions
Indications
    A. Pattern discrimination
    B. Symptomatic or disease indications
Contraindications or prohibitions
Methods of preparation & administration
Modifications

The following questions test all the above areas of Chinese medical knowledge. Because there is a huge amount of material which must be memorized before one can use this system of herbal medicine in a professionally standard and systematic way, the more one rehearses and goes over this information, the sooner one will be able to use it competently in clinical practice.

Chinese herbal medicine is not safe and effective because it is Chinese or because it is herbal. Many of the medicinals used in Chinese herbal medicine do not originate from China and many are not herbal, being animal or mineral in origin. Chinese herbal medicine is the safe and effective medicine it is because of the system or methodology by which it is prescribed. When medicinals are prescribed based on this methodology, one can be sure that the medicinals match the individual patient's pattern, not just their disease.

However, two things make the real-life application of this sophisticated methodology hard to practice. These are 1) the huge number of bits of information which must be memorized to a high degree of precision and 2) a very mature degree of judgment. While this second requirement is almost impossible to teach, the first does yield to frequent repetition. Any and all teaching aids and methodologies which reinforce such frequent repetition help solidify one of the necessary prerequisites of making this system work in clinical practice.

As the reader should quickly see, the correct answer of most of the questions in this book depends on the correct use of technical terminology. The terminology used in this book is based on Nigel Wiseman's *English-Chinese Chinese-English Dictionary of Chinese Medicine*, Hunan Science & Technology Press, Changsha, 1995. For definitions of these terms, students should see Wiseman's *Practical Dictionary of Chinese Medicine*, Paradigm Publications, Brookline, MA, 1998. Chinese medicinals are identified first in Latinate pharmacological nomenclature followed by Pinyin in parentheses. Chinese formulas are identified first by their Pinyin names followed by denotative English language translations in parentheses. An answer key for all these questions is given at the back of this book. An annotated bibliography is also included in the back of this book.

Table of Contents

Exterior-resolving Medicinals (*Jie Biao Yao*)

1. Overuse of acrid, windy, exterior-resolving medicinals may:
   a. Damage yin fluids
   b. Damage qi
   c. Give rise to stirring of wind
   d. Aggravate ascendant liver yang hyperactivity
   e. All of the above

   Answer: ___

2. Herba Ephedrae (*Ma Huang*)'s flavor and nature (*i.e.*, temperature) are:
   a. Acrid, slightly bitter and warm
   b. Acrid, slightly bitter and level (or neutral)
   c. Acrid, slightly sweet and warm
   d. Acrid, salty and cool
   e. Acrid, sweet and cool

   Answer: ___

3. Herba Ephedrae (*Ma Huang*) gathers in or enters which "channels"[1]:
   a. Foot *tai yang* bladder & foot *yang ming* stomach
   b. Foot *tai yin* lung & hand *yang ming* large intestine
   c. Hand *shao yin* heart & hand *tai yang* small intestine
   d. Hand *shao yang* triple burner & foot *shao yin* kidney
   e. Hand *tai yin* lung & foot *tai yang* bladder

   Answer: ___

4. One can reduce Herba Ephedrae (*Ma Huang*)'s effect of resolving the exterior and damaging yin by:
   a. Stir-frying
   b. Mix-frying with honey
   c. Carbonizing
   d. Calcining
   e. Dicing

   Answer: ___

5. Herba Ephedrae (*Ma Huang*) mainly treats:
   a. Wind cold exterior repletion pattern
   b. Wind heat exterior repletion pattern
   c. Exterior vacuity wind cold pattern
   d. Exterior vacuity with wind dampness pattern
   e. None of the above

   Answer: ___

---

[1]   I have placed channels within quotation marks because medicinals do not enter channels per se but affect viscera and bowels.

6. Which of the following medicinals A) resolve the exterior, B) level panting, and C) disinhibit urination:
   a. Herba Elsholtziae (*Xiang Ru*)
   b. Cortex Magnoliae Officinalis (*Hou Po*)
   c. Cortex Radicis Mori Albi (*Sang Bai Pi*)
   d. Herba Ephedrae (*Ma Huang*)
   e. Semen Tinglizi (*Ting Li Zi*)

   Answer: ___

7. Which of the following medicinals is not acrid and warm:
   a. Herba Ephedrae (*Ma Huang*)
   b. Radix Bupleuri (*Chai Hu*)
   c. Ramulus Cinnamomi Cassiae (*Gui Zhi*)
   d. uncooked Rhizoma Zingiberis (*Sheng Jiang*)
   e. Folium Perillae Frutescentis (*Zi Su Ye*)

   Answer: ___

8. Besides resolving the exterior, Ramulus Cinnamomi Cassiae (*Gui Zhi*) also:
   a. Harmonizes the constructive and defensive
   b. Warms the channels and scatters cold
   c. Frees the flow of yang and transforms the qi
   d. Promotes the flow of the blood in its vessels
   e. All of the above

   Answer: ___

9. Which of the following medicinals should be used to treat exterior vacuity with sweating, aversion to wind, and emission of heat (*i.e.*, fever):
   a. Herba Ephedrae (*Ma Huang*)
   b. Radix Astragali Membranacei (*Huang Qi*)
   c. Ramulus Cinnamomi Cassiae (*Gui Zhi*)
   d. Radix Ledebouriellae Divaricatae (*Fang Feng*)
   e. Folium Perillae Frutescentis (*Zi Su Ye*)

   Answer: ___

10. Which of the following medicinals is best for treating painful menstruation and blocked menstruation due to cold stagnating in the channels:
    a. Radix Salviae Miltiorrhizae (*Dan Shen*)
    b. Herba Leonuri Heterophylli (*Yi Mu Cao*)
    c. Tuber Curcumae (*Yu Jin*)
    d. Radix Rubrus Paeoniae Lactiflorae (*Chi Shao*)
    e. Ramulus Cinnamomi Cassiae (*Gui Zhi*)

    Answer: ___

11. Which exterior-resolver A) expels wind, B) out-thrusts rashes, and C) stops bleeding:
    a. Herba Ephedrae (*Ma Huang*)
    b. Folium Perillae Frutescentis (*Zi Su Ye*)
    c. Herba Seu Flos Schizonepetae Tenuifoliae (*Jing Jie Sui*)
    d. Radix Bupleuri (*Chai Hu*)
    e. uncooked Rhizoma Zingiberis (*Sheng Jiang*)

    Answer: ___

12. Folium Perillae Frutescentis (*Zi Su Ye*) can be combined with which of the following medicinals in order to A) resolve the exterior, B) rectify the qi, C) warm the middle, and D) transform turbidity:
    a. Herba Menthae Haplocalycis (*Bo He*)
    b. Herba Agastachis Seu Pogostemi (*Huo Xiang*)
    c. Fructus Amomi (*Sha Ren*)
    d. Fructus Terminaliae Chebulae (*He Zi*)
    e. Radix Bupleuri (*Chai Hu*)

    Answer: ___

13. Folium Perillae Frutescentis (*Zi Su Ye*) enters or gathers in which "channels":
    a. Lung & spleen
    b. Liver & lung
    c. Stomach & large intestine
    d. Spleen & kidney
    e. Heart & lung

    Answer: ___

14. Radix Ledebouriellae Divaricatae (*Fang Feng*) gathers in or enters which of the following "channels":
    a. Foot *tai yang* bladder, foot *jue yin* liver, foot *tai yin* spleen
    b. Foot *tai yang* bladder, foot *jue yin* liver, foot *yang ming* stomach
    c. Hand *tai yang* small intestine, foot *jue yin* liver, foot *tai yin* spleen
    d. Hand *tai yang* small intestine, foot *jue yin* liver, foot *yang ming* stomach
    e. Foot *jue yin* liver, hand and foot *shao yang* gallbladder and triple burner

    Answer: ___

15. Which of the following medicinals is best for external contraction of wind cold with chest oppression due to concomitant qi stagnation:
    a. Herba Seu Flos Schizonepetae Tenuifoliae (*Jing Jie Sui*)
    b. Radix Ledebouriellae Divaricatae (*Fang Feng*)
    c. Folium Perillae Frutescentis (*Zi Su Ye*)
    d. uncooked Rhizoma Zingiberis (*Sheng Jiang*)
    e. Radix Et Rhizoma Notopterygii (*Qiang Huo*)

    Answer: ___

16. Which medicinal guides other medicinals to the *tai yang* and governing vessel:
    a. Rhizoma Coptidis Chinensis (*Huang Lian*)
    b. Rhizoma Anemarrhenae Aspheloidis (*Zhi Mu*)
    c. Radix Et Rhizoma Notopterygii (*Qiang Huo*)
    d. Radix Platycodi Grandiflori (*Jie Geng*)
    e. Radix Angelicae Dahuricae (*Bai Zhi*)

    Answer: ___

17. Which acrid, warm exterior-resolver treats yellow and green nasal discharge due to heat:
    a. Radix Angelicae Dahuricae (*Bai Zhi*)
    b. uncooked Rhizoma Zingiberis (*Sheng Jiang*)
    c. Radix Ledebouriellae Divaricatae (*Fang Feng*)
    d. Ramulus Cinnamomi Cassiae (*Gui Zhi*)
    e. Herba Ephedrae (*Ma Huang*)

    Answer: ___

18. Which acrid, warm exterior-resolver also harmonizes the constructive and defensive and reduces the toxicity of other medicinals:
    a. Herba Asari Cum Radice (*Xi Xin*)
    b. Herba Ledebouriellae Divaricatae (*Fang Feng*)
    c. Herba Seu Flos Schizonepetae Tenuifoliae (*Jing Jie Sui*)
    d. uncooked Rhizoma Zingiberis (*Sheng Jiang*)
    e. Folium Perillae Frutescentis (*Zi Su Ye*)

    Answer: ___

19. Uncooked Rhizoma Zingiberis (*Sheng Jiang*) should be:
    a. Decocted first
    b. Decocted after
    c. Always blast-fried
    d. Decocted with the other medicinals as usual
    e. Only steeped

    Answer: ___

20. Which of the following medicinals is best for external contraction of summerheat with emission of heat, aversion to cold, vomiting, and diarrhea:
    a. uncooked Rhizoma Zingiberis (*Sheng Jiang*)
    b. Herba Elsholtziae (*Xiang Ru*)
    c. Herba Seu Flos Schizonepetae Tenuifoliae (*Jing Jie Sui*)
    d. Folium Perillae Frutescentis (*Zi Su Ye*)
    e. Rhizoma Atractylodis Macrocephalae (*Bai Zhu*)

    Answer: ___

21. Which pair of medicinals treats stomach venter pain, nausea, and vomiting by fortifying the spleen and supplementing the qi:
    a. uncooked Rhizoma Zingiberis (*Sheng Jiang*) & Rhizoma Pinelliae Ternatae (*Ban Xia*)
    b. uncooked Rhizoma Zingiberis (*Sheng Jiang*) & Caulis Bambusae In Taeniis (*Zhu Ru*)
    c. uncooked Rhizoma Zingiberis (*Sheng Jiang*) & Fructus Zizyphi Jujubae (*Da Zao*)
    d. uncooked Rhizoma Zingiberis (*Sheng Jiang*) & Caulis Perillae Frutescentis (*Su Gen*)
    e. uncooked Rhizoma Zingiberis (*Sheng Jiang*) & Rhizoma Coptidis Chinensis (*Huang Lian*)

    Answer: ___

22. Uncooked Rhizoma Zingiberis (*Sheng Jiang*) is best for stopping which pattern of vomiting:
    a. Stomach vacuity
    b. Stomach heat
    c. Qi stagnation
    d. Stomach cold
    e. Food stagnation

    Answer: ___

23. Flos Magnoliae Liliflorae (*Xin Yi Hua*) is commonly combined with which medicinal in order to free the flow of the orifice of the nose:
    a. Fructus Xanthii Sibirici (*Cang Er Zi*)
    b. Bulbus Allii Fistulosi (*Cong Bai*)
    c. Radix Bupleuri (*Chai Hu*)
    d. Radix Scutellariae Baicalensis (*Huang Qin*)
    e. Radix Peucedani (*Qian Hu*)

    Answer: ___

24. Which medicinal dispels wind, scatters cold, and opens the orifice of the nose:
    a. Folium Perillae Frutescentis (*Zi Su Ye*)
    b. uncooked Rhizoma Zingiberis (*Sheng Jiang*)
    c. Radix Et Rhizoma Notoptergyii (*Qiang Huo*)
    d. Flos Magnoliae Liliflorae (*Xin Yi Hua*)
    e. Radix Ledebouriellae Divaricatae (*Fang Feng*)

    Answer: ___

25. In addition to resolving the exterior and clearing heat, Herba Menthae Haplocalycis (*Bo He*):
    a. Clears the head and eyes
    b. Out-thrusts rashes
    c. Courses the liver and resolves depression
    d. A & C
    e. A, B & C

    Answer: __

26. Which is the best medicinal for treating upper body joint and muscular pain due to wind, cold, and dampness:
    a. Radix Et Rhizoma Notoptergyii (*Qiang Huo*)
    b. Ramulus Cinnamomi Cassiae (*Gui Zhi*)
    c. Rhizoma Cibotii Barometsis (*Gou Ji*)
    d. Radix Cyathulae (*Chuan Niu Xi*)
    e. Radix Ledebouriellae Divaricatae (*Fang Feng*)

    Answer: ___

27. Herba Seu Flos Schizonepetae Tenuifoliae (*Jing Jie Sui*) and Radix Ledebouriellae Divaricatae (*Fang Feng*) both:
    a. Dispel wind and resolve the exterior
    b. Dispel wind and eliminate dampness
    c. Dispel wind and resolve tetany
    d. Dispel wind and brighten the eyes
    e. Dispel wind and transform phlegm

    Answer: ___

28. Which medicinal A) resolves the exterior and clears heat, B) disinhibits the throat, C) out-thrusts rashes, and D) moistens the intestines and frees the flow of the stool:
    a. Spica Prunellae Vulgaris (*Xia Ku Cao*)
    b. Fructus Arctii Lappae (*Niu Bang Zi*)
    c. Radix Scutellariae Baicalensis (*Huang Qin*)
    d. Herba Seu Flos Schizonepetae Tenuifoliae (*Jing Jie Sui*)
    e. Rhizoma Cimicifugae (*Sheng Ma*)

    Answer: ___

29. Radix Et Rhizoma Ligustici Chinensis (*Gao Ben*, a.k.a. *Hao Ben*):
    a. Resolves the exterior, opens the orifices, and stops pain
    b. Resolves the exterior, scatters cold, dispels wind, and eliminates dampness
    c. Resolves the exterior, dispels wind, disperses swelling, and stops pain
    d. Resolves the exterior, relaxes tension (cramps and spasms), dispels cold, and stops pain
    e. Dispels wind, eliminates dampness, clears heat, and resolves toxins

    Answer: ___

30. Which medicinal is an exterior-resolver which also extinguishes internally stirring wind:
    a. Lumbricus (*Di Long*)
    b. Buthus Martensis (*Quan Xie*)
    c. Periostracum Cicadae (*Chan Tui*)
    d. Scolopendra Subspinipes (*Wu Gong*)
    e. Ramulus Uncariae Cum Uncis (*Gou Teng*)

    Answer: ___

31. Which exterior-resolving medicinal is effective for treating a *yang ming* headache:
    a. Radix Et Rhizoma Notopterygii (*Qiang Huo*)
    b. Radix Angelicae Dahuricae (*Bai Zhi*)
    c. Radix Ledebouriellae Divaricatae (*Fang Feng*)
    d. Radix Bupleuri (*Chai Hu*)
    e. Rhizoma Atractylodis (*Cang Zhu*)

    Answer: ___

32. Which of the following medicinals is known as "summer *Ma Huang*":
    a. Folium Perillae Frutescentis (*Zi Su Ye*)
    b. Herba Seu Flos Schizonepetae Tenuifoliae (*Jing Jie Sui*)
    c. Herba Eupatorii Fortunei (*Pei Lan*)
    d. Herba Agastachis Seu Pogostemi (*Huo Xiang*)
    e. Herba Elsholtziae (*Xiang Ru*)

    Answer: ___

33. Which of the following medicinals clears the liver and brightens the eyes:
    a. Fructus Mori Albi (*Sang Shen*)
    b. Ramulus Mori Albi (*Sang Zhi*)
    c. Folium Mori Albi (*Sang Ye*)
    d. Ramulus Loranthi Seu Visci (*Sang Ji Sheng*)
    e. Cortex Radicis Mori Albi (*Sang Bai Pi*)

    Answer: ___

34. Which two medicinals can be combined with Folium Mori Albi (*Sang Ye*) when a wind heat external contraction mutually engenders liver heat causing redness and pain in the eyes:
    a. Rhizoma Cimicifugae (*Sheng Ma*) and Radix Puerariae (*Ge Gen*)
    b. Flos Chrysanthemi Morifolii (*Ju Hua*) and Fructus Lycii Chinensis (*Gou Qi Zi*)
    c. Radix Puerariae (*Ge Gen*) and Concha Haliotidis (*Shi Jue Ming*)
    d. Semen Pruni Armeniacae (*Xing Ren*) and Radix Platycodi Grandiflori (*Jie Geng*)
    e. Flos Chrysanthemi Morifolii (*Ju Hua*) and Herba Menthae Haplocalycis (*Bo He*)

    Answer: ___

35. Which exterior-resolver is also an especially good reliever of diarrhea of various types:
    a. uncooked Rhizoma Zingiberis (*Sheng Jiang*)
    b. Radix Ledebouriellae Divaricatae (*Fang Feng*)
    c. Ramulus Cinnamomi Cassiae (*Gui Zhi*)
    d. Radix Puerariae (*Ge Gen*)
    e. Herba Seu Flos Schizonepetae Tenuifoliae (*Jing Jie Sui*)

    Answer: ___

36. Which of the following medicinals dispels wind, stops tetany, and brightens the eyes:
    a. Concha Haliotidis (*Shi Jue Ming*)
    b. Radix Ledebouriellae Divaricatae (*Fang Feng*)
    c. Periostracum Cicadae (*Chan Tui*)
    d. Rhizoma Arisaematis (*Nan Xing*)
    e. Semen Cassiae Torae (*Jue Ming Zi*)

    Answer: ___

37. Which exterior-resolver is most often used in clinical practice to course the liver and rectify the qi:
    a. uncooked Rhizoma Zingiberis (*Sheng Jiang*)
    b. Herba Asari Cum Radice (*Xi Xin*)
    c. Ramulus Cinnamomi Cassiae (*Gui Zhi*)
    d. Radix Bupleuri (*Chai Hu*)
    e. Flos Chrysanthemi Morifolii (*Ju Hua*)

    Answer: ___

38. Which of the following medicinals is best for external contraction of wind heat with cough with phlegm and sore throat:
    a. Semen Praeparatum Sojae (*Dan Dou Chi*)
    b. Fructus Arctii Lappae (*Niu Bang Zi*)
    c. Folium Mori Albi (*Sang Ye*)
    d. Herba Lemnae Seu Spirodelae (*Fu Ping Zi*)
    e. Radix Bupleuri (*Chai Hu*)

    Answer: ___

39. When used to upbear yang, Radix Bupleuri (*Chai Hu*) is usually prescribed:
    a. In a smaller dose than usual
    b. In a larger dose than usual
    c. In its usual dose
    d. Dose does not matter
    e. It's the combination which matters

    Answer: ___

40. Which are more drastic in their exterior-relieving action:
    a. Herba Ephedrae (*Ma Huang*) and Ramulus Cinnamomi Cassiae (*Gui Zhi*)
    b. Radix Ledebouriellae Divaricatae (*Fang Feng*) and Herba Seu Flos Schizonepetae Tenuifoliae (*Jing Jie Sui*)

    Answer: ___

41. Radix Bupleuri (*Chai Hu*):
    a. Emolliates the liver
    b. Courses the liver
    c. Nourishes the liver
    d. Clears the liver
    e. None of the above
    f. All of the above

    Answer: ___

42. Which is the best medicinal for removing screens from the eyes:
    a. Flos Chrysanthemi Morifolii (*Ju Hua*)
    b. Herba Equiseti Hiemalis (*Mu Zei Cao*)
    c. Folium Mori Albi (*Sang Ye*)
    d. Periostracum Cicadae (*Chan Tui*)
    e. Mentha Haplocalycis (*Bo He*)

    Answer: ___

43. Which of the following medicinals is the best for clearing heat:
    a. Folium Mori Albi (*Sang Ye*)
    b. Radix Et Rhizoma Ligustici Chinensis (*Gao Ben*, a.k.a. *Hao Ben*)
    c. Fructus Viticis (*Man Jing Zi*)
    d. Radix Bupleuri (*Chai Hu*)
    e. Periostracum Cicadae (*Chan Tui*)

    Answer: ___

44. Which of the following medicinals is best for an external contraction with emission of heat (or fever) with absence of sweating but headache and stiff neck:
    a. Herba Ephedrae (*Ma Huang*)
    b. Radix Bupleuri (*Chai Hu*)
    c. Ramulus Cinnamomi Cassiae (*Gui Zhi*)
    d. Radix Puerariae (*Ge Gen*)
    e. Rhizoma Cimicifugae (*Sheng Ma*)

    Answer: ___

45. Radix Bupleuri (*Chai Hu*) and Radix Puerariae (*Ge Gen*) both:
    a. Out-thrust rashes
    b. Upbear clear yang
    c. Engender fluids and stop thirst
    d. Course the liver and rectify the qi
    e. Fortify the spleen and stop diarrhea

    Answer: ___

46. Which of the following medicinals A) dispels wind, B) clears heat, and C) resolves toxins:
    a. Rhizoma Cimicifugae (*Sheng Ma*) & Fructus Arctii Lappae (*Niu Bang Zi*)
    b. Flos Lonicerae Japonicae (*Jin Yin Hua*) & Herba Menthae Haplocalycis (*Bo He*)
    c. Flos Chrysanthemi Morifolii (*Ju Hua*) & Periostracum Cicadae (*Chan Tui*)
    d. Herba Menthae Haplocalycis (*Bo He*) & Fructus Forsythiae Suspensae (*Lian Qiao*)
    e. Folium Mori Albi (*Sang Ye*) & Flos Chrysanthemi Morifolii (*Ju Hua*)

    Answer: ___

47. Which of the following medicinals are all acrid, warm exterior-resolvers:
    a. Radix Bupleuri (*Chai Hu*), Folium Perillae Frutescentis (*Zi Su Ye*) & uncooked Rhizoma Zingiberis (*Sheng Jiang*)
    b. Radix Angelicae Dahuricae (*Bai Zhi*), Fructus Arctii Lappae (*Niu Bang Zi*) & Fructus Viticis (*Man Jing Zi*)
    c. Fructus Xanthii Sibirici (*Cang Er Zi*), Radix Et Rhizoma Notopterygii (*Qiang Huo*) & Herba Elsholtziae (*Xiang Ru*)
    d. Herba Menthae Haplocalycis (*Bo He*) & Folium Mori Albi (*Sang Ye*)

    Answer: ___

48. Which medicinals can be used to treat an external contraction of wind cold with absence of sweating but stiff neck:
    a. Herba Ephedrae (*Ma Huang*) & Radix Bupleuri (*Chai Hu*)
    b. Herba Ephedrae (*Ma Huang*) & Ramulus Cinnamomi (*Gui Zhi*)
    c. Ramulus Cinnamomi Cassiae (*Gui Zhi*) & Radix Puerariae (*Ge Gen*)
    d. Radix Puerariae (*Ge Gen*) & Herba Ephedrae (*Ma Huang*)
    e. Radix Et Rhizoma Notopterygii (*Qiang Huo*) & Herba Menthae Haplocalycis (*Bo He*)

    Answer: ___

Heat-clearing Medicinals (*Qing Re Yao*)

49. Medicinals in the heat-clearing category clear which type of heat:
    a. External heat
    b. Internal heat
    c. Neither internal nor external heat
    d. Both internal and external heat

    Answer: ___

50. Gypsum Fibrosum (*Shi Gao*) gathers in or enters which "channels":
    a. Lungs & large intestine
    b. Lungs & heart
    c. Lungs & stomach
    d. Stomach & heart
    e. Stomach & large intestine

    Answer: ___

51. Gypsum Fibrosum (*Shi Gao*)'s functions are to:
    a. Clear heat and drain fire
    b. Clear heat and cool the blood
    c. Clear heat and resolve toxins
    d. Clear heat and eliminate dampness
    e. Clear vacuity heat

    Answer: ___

52. Which of the following medicinals clears heat and drains fire when taken internally and clears heat and heals sores when applied externally:
    a. Gypsum Fibrosum (*Shi Gao*)
    b. Talcum (*Hua Shi*)
    c. Cortex Phellodendri (*Huang Bai*)
    d. Fructus Gardeniae Jasminoidis (*Shan Zhi Zi*)
    e. Radix Trichosanthis Kirlowii (*Tian Hua Fen*)

    Answer: ___

53. Which of the following medicinals is best for toothache with a stomach fire pattern:
    a. uncooked Radix Rehmanniae (*Sheng Di*)
    b. Radix Scrophulariae Ningpoensis (*Xuan Shen*)
    c. Gypsum Fibrosum (*Shi Gao*)
    d. Herba Asari Cum Radice (*Xi Xin*)
    e. Radix Gentianae Scabrae (*Long Dan Cao*)

    Answer: ___

54. Rhizoma Anemarrhenae Aspheloidis (*Zhi Mu*)'s functions are to:
    a. Clear heat and drain fire, enrich yin and moisten dryness
    b. Clear heat and drain fire, resolve vexation and stop thirst
    c. Clear heat and drain fire, cool the blood and resolve toxins
    d. Clear heat and drain fire, resolve toxins and dry dampness
    e. Clear heat and drain fire, engender fluids and stop vomiting

    Answer: ___

55. When Rhizoma Anemarrhenae Aspheloidis (*Zhi Mu*) is used to clear heat and drain fire in the case of yin vacuity/vacuity heat conditions, it is most commonly combined with:
    a. Radix Scutellariae Baicalensis (*Huang Qin*)
    b. Cortex Phellodendri (*Huang Bai*)
    c. Fructus Gardeniae Jasminoidis (*Shan Zhi Zi*)
    d. Rhizoma Coptidis Chinensis (*Huang Lian*)
    e. Radix Et Rhizoma Rhei (*Da Huang*)

    Answer: ___

56. To increase Rhizoma Anemarrhenae Aspheloidis (*Zhi Mu*)'s downbearing nature, it can be:
    a. Stir-fried in alcohol
    b. Stir-fried in vinegar
    c. Stir-fried in saltwater
    d. Mix-fried with honey
    e. Used uncooked

    Answer: ___

57. Which medicinal clears both replete and vacuity heat:
    a. Radix Scutellariae Baicalensis (*Huang Qin*)
    b. Gypsum Fibrosum (*Shi Gao*)
    c. Rhizoma Anemarrhenae Aspheloidis (*Zhi Mu*)
    d. Radix Sophorae Flavescentis (*Ku Shen*)
    e. Fructus Gardeniae Jasminoidis (*Shan Zhi Zi*)

    Answer: ___

58. In order to clear heat and resolve depression, cool the blood and stop bleeding, choose:
    a. Rhizoma Imperatae Cylindricae (*Bai Mao Gen*)
    b. Folium Lophatheri Gracilis (*Dan Zhu Ye*)
    c. Spica Prunellae Vulgaris (*Xia Ku Cao*)
    d. Gypsum Fibrosum (*Shi Gao*)
    e. Fructus Gardeniae Jasminoidis (*Shan Zhi Zi*)

    Answer: ___

59. Which of the following medicinals A) clears heat from the qi division with high fever and irritability and B) cools the blood and stops bleeding:
    a. Fructus Gardeniae Jasminoidis (*Shan Zhi Zi*)
    b. Radix Trichosanthis Kirlowii (*Tian Hua Fen*)
    c. Gypsum Fibrosum (*Shi Gao*)
    d. Rhizoma Anemarrhenae Aspheloidis (*Zhi Mu*)
    e. Rhizoma Phragmitis Communis (*Lu Gen*)

    Answer: ___

60. Spica Prunella Vulgaris (*Xia Ku Cao*):
    a. Clears heat and eliminates dampness
    b. Clears heat and scatters nodulations
    c. Clears heat and moistens dryness
    d. Clears heat and cools the blood
    e. None of the above

    Answer: ___

61. Which of the following medicinals A) clears heat, B) engenders fluids, and C) treats lung abscess:
    a. Rhizoma Phragmitis Communis (*Lu Gen*)
    b. Herba Houttuyniae Cordatae Cum Radice (*Yu Xing Cao*)
    c. Folium Lophatheri Gracilis (*Dan Zhu Ye*)
    d. Fructus Trichosanthis Kirlowii (*Tian Hua Fen*)
    e. Radix Platycodi Grandiflori (*Jie Geng*)

    Answer: ___

62. Cornu _____ can be substituted for Cornu Rhinocerotis (*Xi Jiao*):
    a. Caprae (*Yang Jiao*)
    b. Cervi (*Lu Jiao*)
    c. Bubali (*Shui Niu Jiao*)
    d. Copia (*Yu No Jiao*)
    e. Canis (*Kou Jiao*)

    Answer: ___

63. Which of the following medicinals does not clear heat and dry dampness:
    a. Rhizoma Coptidis Chinensis (*Huang Lian*)
    b. Radix Sophorae Flavescentis (*Ku Shen*)
    c. Cortex Phellodendri (*Huang Bai*)
    d. Folium Lophatheri Gracilis (*Dan Zhu Ye*)
    e. Radix Scutellariae Baicalensis (*Huang Qin*)

    Answer: ___

64. Which Rehmannia (*Di Huang*) should you use if you want to cool the blood:
    a. uncooked Radix Rehmanniae (*Sheng Di*)
    b. cooked Radix Rehmanniae (*Shu Di*)

    Answer: ___

65. Which of the following medicinals is best for damp heat in the stomach and intestines causing diarrhea, dysentery, and vomiting:
    a. Rhizoma Coptidis Chinensis (*Huang Lian*)
    b. Radix Scutellariae Baicalensis (*Huang Qin*)
    c. Cortex Phellodendri (*Huang Bai*)
    d. Fructus Gardeniae Jasminoidis (*Shan Zhi Zi*)
    e. Radix Gentianae Scabrae (*Long Dan Cao*)

    Answer: ___

66. Cortex Radicis Moutan (*Dan Pi*) is added to yin-supplementing formulas, such as *Liu Wei Di Huang Wan* (Six Flavors Rehmannia Pills), because:
    a. It clears heat and cools the blood
    b. It clears vacuity heat
    c. It quickens the blood and dispels stasis
    d. It drains ascending liver fire
    e. All of the above

    Answer: ___

67. Cortex Radicis Lycii Chinensis (*Di Gu Pi*) clears what kind of heat:
    a. Replete heat
    b. Vacuity heat
    c. Damp heat
    d. Summerheat
    e. Heat toxins

    Answer: ___

68. Radix Scutellariae Baicalensis (*Huang Qin*):
    a. Easily damages stomach qi
    b. Does not easily damage stomach qi

    Answer: ___

69. Radix Scutellariae Baicalensis (*Huang Qin*) gathers in or enters which "channels":
    a. Heart, spleen, stomach, and large intestine
    b. Heart, lungs, spleen, and large intestine
    c. Lungs, stomach, large intestine, gallbladder
    d. Lungs, liver, gallbladder, and bladder
    e. All of the above

    Answer: ___

70. Which medicinal clears heat, eliminates dampness, and quiets the fetus:
    a. Rhizoma Coptidis Chinensis (*Huang Lian*)
    b. Radix Scutellariae Baicalensis (*Huang Qin*)
    c. Cortex Phellodendri (*Huang Bai*)
    d. Fructus Gardeniae Jasminoidis (*Shan Zhi Zi*)
    e. Radix Et Rhizoma Rhei (*Da Huang*)

    Answer: ___

71. Which of the following medicinals is best for lung heat cough:
    a. Radix Scutellariae Baicalensis (*Huang Qin*)
    b. Rhizoma Coptidis Chinensis (*Huang Lian*)
    c. Fructus Gardeniae Jasminoidis (*Shan Zhi Zi*)
    d. Cortex Phellodendri (*Huang Bai*)
    e. Radix Gentianae Scabrae (*Long Dan Cao*)

    Answer: ___

72. Which of the following medicinals is best for clearing heat, eliminating dampness, and draining liver fire:
    a. Semen Cassiae Torae (*Jue Ming Zi*)
    b. Radix Scutellariae Baicalensis (*Huang Qin*)
    c. Radix Gentianae Scabrae (*Long Dan Cao*)
    d. Semen Celosiae Cristatae (*Qing Xian Zi*)
    e. Cortex Phellodendri (*Huang Bai*)

    Answer: ___

73. Rhizoma Coptidis Chinensis (*Huang Lian*) gathers in or enters which "channels":
    a. Heart, stomach, large intestine, and liver
    b. Heart, spleen, stomach, and liver
    c. Heart, spleen, liver, and kidneys
    d. Stomach, large intestine, gallbladder, and bladder
    e. None of the above

    Answer: ___

74. If there is lack of interconnection between the heart and kidneys, Rhizoma Coptidis Chinensis (*Huang Lian*) can be combined with:
    a. Fructus Gardeniae Jasminoidis (*Shan Zhi Zi*)
    b. Cortex Phellodendri (*Huang Bai*)
    c. Cortex Cinnamomi Cassiae (*Rou Gui*)
    d. Radix Panacis Ginseng (*Ren Shen*)
    e. Radix Angelicae Sinensis (*Dang Gui*)

    Answer: ___

75. Rhizoma Coptidis Chinensis (*Huang Lian*) should be:
    a. Decocted after
    b. Decocted first
    c. Decocted with the other medicinals as usual
    d. Always used uncooked
    e. Never used uncooked

    Answer: ___

76. Radix Gentianae Scabrae (*Long Dan Cao*) is commonly used to treat which of the following conditions:
    a. Acid eructations caused by stomach heat
    b. Dysentery caused by heat toxins
    c. Welling abscesses caused by heat toxins
    d. Abnormal vaginal discharge and external vaginal itching due to damp heat
    e. Damage and detriment due to scalding and burns

    Answer: ___

77. Cortex Phellodendri (*Huang Bai*):
    a. Clears replete heat above and depressive heat below
    b. Clears vacuity heat above and damp heat below
    c. Clears heat and resolves toxins
    d. A & C
    e. B & C

    Answer: ___

78. Radix Gentianae Scabrae (*Long Dan Cao*):
    a. Easily damages the stomach qi
    b. Seldom damages the stomach qi

    Answer: ___

79. Radix Sophorae Flavescentis (*Ku Shen*) mainly treats:
    a. Coughs and skin diseases
    b. Skin diseases and eye complaints
    c. Eye complaints and coughs
    d. Skin diseases and genital sores
    e. Mental-emotional disturbances and tremors

    Answer: ___

80. In real-life clinical practice, Cortex Fraxini (*Qin Pi*) is primarily combined with Radix Pulsatillae Chinensis (*Bai Tou Weng*) to treat:
    a. Phlegm heat cough
    b. Damp heat strangury
    c. Damp heat diarrhea and dysentery
    d. Cold damp diarrhea and dysentery
    e. Unstoppable, enduring diarrhea and dysentery

    Answer: ___

81. Flos Lonicerae Japonicae (*Jin Yin Hua*) is most commonly combined with what other heat-clearing, toxin-resolving medicinal:
    a. Cortex Phellodendri (*Huang Bai*)
    b. Fructus Forsythiae Suspensae (*Lian Qiao*)
    c. Rhizoma Picrorrhizae (*Hu Huang Lian*)
    d. Carapax Amydae Sinensis (*Bei Jia*)
    e. Radix Scrophulariae Ningpoensis (*Xuan Shen*)

    Answer: ___

82. Flos Lonicerae Japonicae (*Jin Yin Hua*)'s flavor and nature (*i.e.*, temperature) are:
    a. Acrid, bitter & slightly cold
    b. Bitter & cold
    c. Sour & cold
    d. Sweet & cold
    e. Acrid and slightly cold

    Answer: ___

83. Which heat-clearing, toxin-resolving medicinal is often taken in China for the prevention of viral epidemics:
    a. Fructus Forsythiae Suspensae (*Lian Qiao*)
    b. Radix Puerariae (*Ge Gen*)
    c. Radix Isatidis Seu Baphicacanthi (*Ban Lan Gen*)
    d. Flos Lonicerae Japonicae (*Jin Yin Hua*)
    e. Chinese medicinals should not be taken preventively

    Answer: ___

84. Herba Taraxaci Mongolici Cum Radice (*Pu Gong Ying*):
    a. Clears heat and resolves toxins
    b. Courses the liver and resolves depression
    c. Disperses swelling and scatters nodulations
    d. Frees the flow of milk
    e. All of the above

    Answer: ___

85. Calculus Bovis (*Niu Huang*)'s functions are to:
    a. Subdue the liver and extinguish wind, clear heat and resolve toxins
    b. Extinguish wind and resolve tetany, wash away phlegm and open the orifices
    c. Clear heat and extinguish wind, level panting and free the flow of the network vessels
    d. Extinguish wind and level the liver
    e. Extinguish wind and resolve tetany, dispel wind and stop pain

    Answer: ___

86. Herba Patriniae Heterophyllae Cum Radice (*Bai Jiang Cao*) is especially good for treating ____ lower abdominal pain due to damp heat stasis and stagnation:
    a. right-sided
    b. left-sided
    c. center

    Answer: ___

87. Which medicinal is known to be empirically especially effective when there is cough with thick, greenish yellow phlegm:
    a. Radix Platycodi Grandiflori (*Jie Geng*)
    b. Herba Houttuyniae Cordatae Cum Radice (*Yu Xing Cao*)
    c. Radix Scutellariae Baicalensis (*Huang Qin*)
    d. Bulbus Fritillariae Cirrhosae (*Chuan Bei Mu*)
    e. Pericarpium Citri Reticulatae (*Chen Pi*)

    Answer: ___

88. Besides Herba Patriniae Heterophyllae Cum Radice (*Bai Jiang Cao*), which other medicinal is especially good for damp heat stasis and stagnation:
    a. Herba Taraxaci Mongolici Cum Radice (*Pu Gong Ying*)
    b. Herba Violae Yedoensitis Cum Radice (*Zi Hua Di Ding*)
    c. Radix Isatidis Seu Baphicacanthi (*Ban Lan Gen*)
    d. Fructus Gardeniae Jasminoidis (*Shan Zhi Zi*)
    e. Caulis Sargentodoxae (*Hong Teng*)

    Answer: ___

89. During a warm disease, which is the best of the following medicinals when heat has entered the constructive division with dry mouth and a red tongue:
    a. Cornu Rhinocerotis (*Xi Jiao*)
    b. uncooked Radix Rehmanniae (*Sheng Di*)
    c. Cortex Radicis Moutan (*Dan Pi*)
    d. Rhizoma Anemarrhenae Aspheloidis (*Zhi Mu*)
    e. Fructus Gardeniae Jasminoidis (*Shan Zhi Zi*)

    Answer: ___

90. Which of the following medicinals A) cools the blood and stops bleeding and B) quickens the blood and dispels stasis:
    a. uncooked Radix Rehmanniae (*Sheng Di*)
    b. Rhizoma Imperatae Cylindricae (*Bai Mao Gen*)
    c. Radix Rubrus Paeoniae Lactiflorae (*Chi Shao*)
    d. Radix Pseudoginseng (*Tian San Qi*)
    e. Cortex Radicis Lycii Chinensis (*Di Gu Pi*)

    Answer: ___

91. Radix Scrophulariae Ningpoensis (*Xuan Shen*)'s flavor and nature (*i.e.*, temperature) are:
    a. Sweet & cold
    b. Bitter & cold
    c. Salty & cold
    d. Salty, sweet & cold
    e. Bitter, sweet, salty & cold

    Answer: ___

92. Radix Scrophulariae Ningpoensis (*Xuan Shen*) can be used in all of the following conditions except:
    a. Gangrene of the extremities
    b. During a blood heat division warm disease with skin rash
    c. Phlegm and heat mutually binding to form nodulations
    d. Severe yin vacuity with vacuity fire causing sore throat
    e. Evil heat exuberance with high fever, thirst, irritability, and a surging pulse

    Answer: ___

93. Which of the following medicinals is best in cases of severe heat toxins, inability of rashes to be outthrust, and dark, purple-colored rashes:
    a. Fructus Arctii Lappae (*Niu Bang Zi*)
    b. Rhizoma Cimicifugae (*Sheng Ma*)
    c. Flos Carthami Tinctorii (*Hong Hua*)
    d. Radix Rubrus Paeoniae Lactiflorae (*Chi Shao*)
    e. Radix Lithospermi Seu Arnebiae (*Zi Cao*)

    Answer: ___

94. Which of the following medicinals resolves toxins, eliminates dampness, and disinhibits the joints:
    a. Radix Clematidis Chinensis (*Wei Ling Xian*)
    b. Rhizoma Smilacis Glabrae (*Tu Fu Ling*)
    c. Herba Houttuyniae Cordatae Cum Radice (*Yu Xing Cao*)
    d. Semen Plantaginis (*Che Qian Zi*)
    e. Radix Rubrus Paeoniae Lactiflorae (*Chi Shao*)

    Answer: ___

95. What clearing heat and resolving summerheat medicinal also upbears clear yang and stops bleeding:
    a. Semen Phaseoli Munginis (*Lu Dou*)
    b. Semen Dolichoris Lablab (*Bai Bian Dou*)
    c. Herba Artemisiae Apiaceae (*Qing Hao*)
    d. Folium Nelumbinis Nuciferae (*He Ye*)
    e. Rhizoma Cimicifugae (*Sheng Ma*)

    Answer: ___

96. In order to fortify the spleen, eliminate dampness, and stop diarrhea without damaging yin fluids, Semen Dolichoris Lablab (*Bai Bian Dou*) is commonly combined with:
    a. Radix Dioscoreae Oppositae (*Shan Yao*)
    b. Rhizoma Atractylodis (*Cang Zhu*)
    c. Rhizoma Atractylodis Macrocephalae (*Bai Zhu*)
    d. Fructus Cardamomi (*Bai Dou Kou*)
    e. Fructus Amomi (*Sha Ren*)

    Answer: ___

97. Which of the following medicinals is commonly used to treat damp heat skin lesions:
    a. Cortex Radicis Dictamni Dasycarpi (*Bai Xian Pi*)
    b. Folium Daqingye (*Da Qing Ye*)
    c. Rhizoma Belamcandae (*She Gan*)
    d. Rhizoma Bletillae Striatae (*Bai Ji*)
    e. uncooked Radix Rehmanniae (*Sheng Di*)

    Answer: ___

98. Which of the following medicinals not only cools the blood and abates bone-steaming emission of heat but also clears and drains lung heat:
    a. Cortex Phellodendri (*Huang Bai*)
    b. Rhizoma Anemarrhenae Aspheloidis (*Zhi Mu*)
    c. Cortex Radicis Lycii Chinensis (*Di Gu Pi*)
    d. Radix Stellariae Dichotomae (*Yin Chai Hu*)
    e. Fructus Gardeniae Jasminoidis (*Shan Zhi Zi*)

    Answer: ___

99. Both Cortex Radicis Lycii Chinensis (*Di Gu Pi*) and Cortex Radicis Moutan (*Dan Pi*):
    a. Clear heat and resolve toxins
    b. Clear vacuity heat
    c. Quicken the blood and dispel stasis
    d. Clear heat and dry dampness
    e. All of the above

    Answer: ___

100. Both Radix Scrophulariae Ningpoensis (*Xuan Shen*) and uncooked Radix Rehmanniae (*Sheng Di*) treat:
    a. Heat evils in the constructive division with generalized heat, dry mouth, and a red tongue
    b. Welling abscesses, scrofulous lumps, and sore throat
    c. Blood vacuity causing internal heat and painful menstruation
    d. Damp heat pattern jaundice
    e. Heat evils in the qi division with thirst and irritability

    Answer: ___

101. Both Radix Gentianae Scabrae (*Long Dan Cao*) and Radix Sophorae Flavescentis (*Ku Shen*):
    a. Clear heat and drain fire
    b. Clear heat and cool the blood
    c. Clear heat and resolve toxins
    d. Clear heat and eliminate dampness
    e. Clear vacuity heat

    Answer: ___

102. Which two medicinals clear heat and cool the blood, nourish yin and engender fluids:
    a. Cornu Rhinocerotis (*Xi Jiao*) & uncooked Radix Rehmanniae (*Sheng Di*)
    b. Radix Scrophulariae Ningpoensis (*Xuan Shen*) & Cortex Radicis Moutan (*Dan Pi*)
    c. Radix Glehniae Littoralis (*Sha Shen*) & Radix Rubrus Paeoniae Lactiflorae (*Chi Shao*)
    d. Radix Scrophulariae Ningpoensis (*Xuan Shen*) & uncooked Radix Rehmanniae (*Sheng Di*)
    e. Cornu Rhinocerotis (*Xi Jiao*) & Cortex Radicis Lycii Chinensis (*Di Gu Pi*)

    Answer: ___

103. Which two medicinals clear lung and stomach heat:
    a. Cortex Phellodendri (*Huang Bai*) & Folium Lophatheri Gracilis (*Dan Zhu Ye*)
    b. Rhizoma Phragmitis Communis (*Lu Gen*) & Rhizoma Anemarrhenae Aspheloidis (*Zhi Mu*)
    c. Gypsum Fibrosum (*Shi Gao*) & Spica Prunellae Vulgaris (*Xia Ku Cao*)
    d. Radix Trichosanthis Kirlowii (*Tian Hua Fen*) & Radix Gentianae Scabrae (*Long Dan Cao*)
    e. Radix Scutellariae Baicalensis (*Huang Qin*) & Radix Rubrus Paeoniae Lactiflorae (*Chi Shao*)

    Answer: ___

104. Which two medicinals clear heat and cool the blood, quicken the blood and dispel stasis:
    a. Flos Lonicerae Japonicae (*Jin Yin Hua*) & Fructus Forsythiae Suspensae (*Lian Qiao*)
    b. Cornu Rhinocerotis (*Xi Jiao*) & uncooked Radix Rehmanniae (*Sheng Di*)
    c. Radix Rubrus Paeoniae Lactiflorae (*Chi Shao*) & Cortex Radicis Moutan (*Da Pi*)
    d. Rhizoma Sparganii (*San Leng*) & Rhizoma Curcumae Zedoariae (*E Zhu*)
    e. Semen Coicis Lachryma-jobi (*Yi Yi Ren*) & Herba Cephalanoploris Segeti (*Xiao Ji*)

    Answer: ___

105. Both Herba Portulacae Oleraceae (*Ma Chi Xian*) and Radix Pulsatillae Chinensis (*Bai Tou Weng*):
    a. Clear heat, resolve toxins, and brighten the eyes
    b. Clear heat, resolve toxins, and treat dysentery
    c. Clear heat, resolve toxins, and disinhibit the throat
    d. Clear heat, resolve toxins, and treat lung abscesses
    e. None of the above

    Answer: ___

106. Both Spica Prunellae Vulgaris (*Xia Ku Cao*) and Radix Gentianae Scabrae (*Long Dan Cao*):
    a. Clear the liver
    b. Clear the heart
    c. Clear the stomach
    d. Clear the large intestine
    e. Clear the lungs

    Answer: ___

Downward Precipitating Medicinals (*Xia Xie Yao*)

107. If one wants to make use of Radix Et Rhizoma Rhei (*Da Huang*)'s downward precipitating, bitter, and cold function and nature, it should be:
    a. Decocted with the other medicinals as usual
    b. Decocted in advance
    c. Decocted after
    d. Stir-fried in alcohol
    e. Mix-fried in honey

    Answer: ___

108. When treating damp heat pattern jaundice, one should use:
    a. Mirabilitum (*Mang Xiao*)
    b. Radix Et Rhizoma Rhei (*Da Huang*)
    c. Folium Sennae (*Fan Xie Ye*)
    d. Semen Pruni (*Yu Li Ren*)
    e. Semen Cannabis Sativae (*Huo Ma Ren*)

    Answer: ___

109. Which precipitating medicinal enters the blood division:
    a. Mirabilitum (*Mang Xiao*)
    b. Radix Et Rhizoma Rhei (*Da Huang*)
    c. Folium Sennae (*Fan Xie Ye*)
    d. Semen Pruni (*Yu Li Ren*)
    e. Semen Cannabis Sativae (*Huo Ma Ren*)

    Answer: ___

110. Alcohol stir-fried Radix Et Rhizoma Rhei (*Da Huang*) is best for treating:
    a. Blood stasis
    b. Heat accumulation constipation
    c. Welling abscesses due to heat toxins
    d. Damp heat dysentery
    e. Blood heat bleeding

    Answer: ___

111. Radix Et Rhizoma Rhei (*Da Huang*) mainly treats:
    a. Heat accumulation constipation
    b. Cold accumulation constipation
    c. Blood vacuity constipation
    d. Fluid dryness constipation
    e. Yang vacuity constipation

    Answer: ___

112. Mirabilitum (*Mang Xiao*) should be:
    a. Decocted with the other medicinals as usual
    b. Decocted first
    c. Decocted after
    d. Dissolved in the strained decoction

    Answer: ___

113. Which of the following medicinals A) precipitates, B) softens the hard, and C) clears heat:
    a. Radix Et Rhizoma Rhei (*Da Huang*)
    b. Mirabilitum (*Mang Xiao*)
    c. Spica Prunellae Vulgaris (*Xia Ku Cao*)
    d. Concha Ostreae (*Mu Li*)
    e. Radix Scrophulariae Ningpoensis (*Xuan Shen*)

    Answer: ___

114. Semen Cannabis Sativae (*Huo Ma Ren*) is most appropriate for:
    a. Fluid dryness constipation
    b. Qi vacuity constipation
    c. Qi stagnation constipation
    d. Blood stasis constipation
    e. Yang vacuity constipation

    Answer: ___

115. Which is the mildest precipitating medicinal which also treats intestinal worms and food stagnation:
    a. Radix Euphorbiae Kansui (*Gan Sui*)
    b. Radix Euphorbiae Knoxiae (*Da Ji*)
    c. Flos Daphnes Genkwae (*Yuan Hua*)
    d. Semen Pharbiditis (*Qian Niu Zi*)

    Answer: ___

116. Which of the following medicinals A) precipitates and frees the flow of the stools and B) clears the liver and kills worms:
    a. Fructus Quisqualis Indicae (*Shi Jun Zi*)
    b. Herba Aloes (*Lu Hui*)
    c. Cortex Meliae Azardachis (*Ku Lian Gen*)
    d. Folium Sennae (*Fan Xie Ye*)
    e. Fructificatio Polypori Mylittae (*Lei Wan*)

    Answer: ___

117. Semen Pruni (*Yu Li Ren*) not only moistens the intestines and frees the flow of the stools but also:
    a. Eliminates dampness and recedes jaundice
    b. Disinhibits urination and disperses swelling
    c. Softens the hard and dispels stasis
    d. Clears the liver and brightens the eyes
    e. Dispels wind and stops pain

    Answer: ___

118. Which of the following medicinals is very hot and very poisonous:
    a. Herba Euphorbiae Pekinensis (*Da Ji*)
    b. Radix Phytolaccae (*Shang Lu*)
    c. Semen Crotonis Tiglii (*Ba Dou*)
    d. Herba Aloes (*Lu Hui*)
    e. Semen Cannabis Sativae (*Huo Ma Ren*)

    Answer: ___

119. If, after taking Semen Crotonis Tiglii (*Ba Dou*), there is enduring diarrhea, this can be relieved by taking:
    a. Warm water
    b. Cold rice porridge
    c. Honey
    d. Uncooked ginger soup
    e. Licorice soup

    Answer: ___

120. Radix Euphorbiae Kansui (*Gan Sui*), Herba Euphorbiae Pekinensis (*Da Ji*), and Flos Daphnes Genkwae (*Yuan Hua*) all treat:
    a. Traumatic injuries and pain
    b. Wind damp impediment conditions
    c. Poisonous snake bites
    d. Water swelling and urinary strangury due to spleen vacuity
    e. Abdominal ascites and fluid accumulation in the chest and abdomen

    Answer: ___

121. Which of the following medicinals can be used to treat blood stasis pattern blocked menstruation or amenorrhea:
    a. Radix Et Rhizoma Rhei (*Da Huang*)
    b. Mirabilitum (*Mang Xiao*)
    c. Radix Euphorbiae Kansui (*Gan Sui*)
    d. Semen Crotonis Tiglii (*Ba Dou*)
    e. Semen Pruni (*Yu Li Ren*)

    Answer: ___

Damp-dispelling Medicinals (*Qu Shi Yao*)

122. Which type of Poria (*Fu Ling*) is best when there is damp heat:
    a. White Sclerotium Poriae Cocos (*Bai Fu Ling*)
    b. Red Sclerotium Poriae Cocos (*Chi Fu Ling*)
    c. Sclerotium Pararadicis Poriae Cocos (*Fu Shen*)
    d. Cortex Sclerotii Poriae Cocos (*Fu Ling Pi*)

    Answer: ___

123. What are the flavor and nature (*i.e.*, temperature) of Sclerotium Poriae Cocos (*Fu Ling*):
    a. Sweet, acrid & cold
    b. Sweet, sour & warm
    c. Salty, acrid & level (*i.e.*, neutral)
    d. Sweet, bland & level (*i.e.*, neutral)
    e. Sweet, bitter & cool

    Answer: ___

124. Which function does Sclerotium Poriae Cocos (*Fu Ling*) not do:
    a. Seeps dampness and disinhibits urination
    b. Fortifies the spleen and harmonizes the middle
    c. Courses the liver and rectifies the qi
    d. Eliminates dampness and transforms phlegm
    e. Calms the heart and quiets the spirit

    Answer: ___

125. Which symptoms does Sclerotium Poriae Cocos (*Fu Ling*) not treat:
    a. Edema & dysuria
    b. Phlegm obstruction causing nausea, heart palpitations, and cough
    c. Fatigue, lack of appetite, and diarrhea due to spleen vacuity
    d. Heart palpitations & insomnia
    e. Vexatious thirst due to summerheat and diarrhea due to damp heat

    Answer: ___

126. Which of the following medicinals resolves the exterior and promotes perspiration, dries dampness and fortifies the spleen:
    a. Rhizoma Atractylodis (*Cang Zhu*)
    b. Radix Et Rhizoma Notopterygii (*Qiang Huo*)
    c. Herba Elsholtziae (*Xiang Ru*)
    d. Fructus Amomi (*Sha Ren*)
    e. Fructus Xanthii Sibirici (*Cang Er Zi*)

    Answer: ___

127. Which of the following not only dries dampness and fortifies the spleen but also dispels wind dampness:
    a. Pericarpium Citri Reticulatae (*Chen Pi*)
    b. Sclerotium Poriae Cocos (*Fu Ling*)
    c. Rhizoma Atractylodis (*Cang Zhu*)
    d. Rhizoma Atractylodis Macrocephalae (*Bai Zhu*)
    e. Cortex Magnoliae Officinalis (*Hou Po*)

    Answer: ___

128. Semen Coicis Lachryma-jobi (*Yi Yi Ren*) is unique because it both:
    a. Clears heat and cools the blood
    b. Fortifies the spleen and clears and eliminates damp heat
    c. Dispels dampness and moistens dryness
    d. Resolves and secures the exterior
    e. Clears heat and scatters cold

    Answer: ___

129. When used to clear heat and eliminate dampness, Semen Coicis Lachryma-jobi (*Yi Yi Ren*) should be used:
    a. Uncooked
    b. Stir-fried
    c. Mix-fried
    d. Carbonized
    e. Stir-fried in vinegar

    Answer: ___

130. Which medicinal treats both lung and intestinal abscesses:
    a. Herba Houttuyniae Cordatae Cum Radice (*Yu Xing Cao*)
    b. Semen Coicis Lachryma-jobi (*Yi Yi Ren*)
    c. Radix Platycodi Grandiflori (*Jie Geng*)
    d. Herba Patriniae Heterophyllae Cum Radice (*Bai Jiang Cao*)
    e. Cortex Radicis Moutan (*Dan Pi*)

    Answer: ___

131. Cortex Magnoliae Officinalis (*Hou Po*)'s flavor and nature (*i.e.*, temperature) are:
    a. Bitter, acrid & warm
    b. Sweet, bitter & warm
    c. Bitter, acrid & cold
    d. Sour, bitter & warm
    e. Acrid, sweet & cool

    Answer: ___

132. Which of the following medicinals can be used to treat damp obstruction causing qi stagnation:
    a. Folium Perillae Frutescentis (*Zi Su Ye*)
    b. Rhizoma Atractylodis (*Cang Zhu*)
    c. Radix Auklandiae Lappae (*Mu Xiang*)
    d. Cortex Magnoliae Officinalis (*Hou Po*)
    e. None of the above

    Answer: ___

133. Rhizoma Dioscoreae Hypoglaucae (*Bei Xie*) is commonly combined with _____ for turbid urine:
    a. Radix Scutellariae Baicalensis (*Huang Qin*)
    b. Rhizoma Coptidis Chinensis (*Huang Lian*)
    c. Radix Et Rhizoma Rhei (*Da Huang*)
    d. Fructus Tribuli Terrestris (*Bai Ji Li*)
    e. Rhizoma Acori Graminei (*Shi Chang Pu*)

    Answer: ___

134. Fructus Cardamomi (*Bai Dou Kou*):
    a. Dries dampness, rectifies the qi, warms the middle burner, and stops diarrhea
    b. Dries dampness, rectifies the qi, warms the middle burner, and stops vomiting
    c. Dries dampness, rectifies the qi, warms the middle burner, and stops vaginal discharge
    d. Dries dampness, rectifies the qi, disperses swelling, and levels panting
    e. Dries dampness, clears summerheat, and stops vomiting

    Answer: ___

135. Which of the following medicinals dries dampness, rectifies the qi, and quiets the fetus:
    a. Herba Eupatorii Fortunei (*Pei Lan*)
    b. Herba Agastachis Seu Pogostemi (*Huo Xiang*)
    c. Cortex Magnoliae Officinalis (*Hou Po*)
    d. Fructus Alpiniae Oxyphyllae (*Yi Zhi Ren*)
    e. Fructus Amomi (*Sha Ren*)

    Answer: ___

136. Fructus Amomi (*Sha Ren*) mainly treats:
    a. Diarrhea due to summerheat dampness
    b. Heat toxins dysentery
    c. Spleen cold diarrhea
    d. Damp heat diarrhea
    e. Food stagnation diarrhea

    Answer: ___

137. Which is the best medicinal for aversion to cold, emission of heat, chest oppression, vomiting, and diarrhea with thick, turbid tongue fur:
    a. Herba Elsholtziae (*Xiang Ru*)
    b. Rhizoma Atractylodis (*Cang Zhu*)
    c. Herba Agastachis Seu Pogostemi (*Huo Xiang*)
    d. Folium Perillae Frutescentis (*Zi Su Ye*)
    e. Herba Eupatorii Fortunei (*Pei Lan*)

    Answer: ___

138. Which medicinal A) eliminates dampness and clears summerheat and B) treats profuse saliva and a sweet, slimy taste in the mouth:
    a. Fructus Alpiniae Oxyphyllae (*Yi Zhi Ren*)
    b. Fructus Amomi (*Sha Ren*)
    c. Cortex Magnoliae Officinalis (*Hou Po*)
    d. Fructus Cardamomi (*Bai Dou Kou*)
    e. Herba Eupatorii Fortunei (*Pei Lan*)

    Answer: ___

139. Which medicinals A) eliminate dampness and B) clear summerheat:
    a. Herba Agastachis Seu Pogostemi (*Huo Xiang*) & Herba Eupatorii Fortunei (*Pei Lan*)
    b. Rhizoma Atractylodis (*Cang Zhu*) & Cortex Magnoliae Officinalis *(Hou Po)*
    c. Fructus Amomi (*Sha Ren*) & Fructus Cardamomi (*Bai Dou Kou*)
    d. Pericarpium Citri Reticulatae (*Chen Pi*) & Pericarpium Citri Reticulatae Viride (*Qing Pi*)
    e. Radix Scutellariae Baicalensis (*Huang Qin*) & Rhizoma Coptidis Chinensis (*Huang Lian*)

    Answer: ___

140. Which symptoms can be treated by either Fructus Amomi (*Sha Ren*) or Fructus Cardamomi (*Bai Dou Kou*):
    a. Spleen yang vacuity diarrhea
    b. Vomiting during pregnancy
    c. Liver depression/depressive heat fetal stirring restlessness
    d. Damp obstruction causing qi stagnation with disharmony of the spleen and stomach
    e. All of the above

    Answer: ___

141. Which of the following medicinals A) treats malaria-like (*nue*) conditions as well as B) warms the middle and dries dampness:
    a. Herba Artemisiae Apiaceae (*Qing Hao*)
    b. Radix Dichroae Febrifugae (*Chang Shan*)
    c. Semen Plantaginis (*Che Qian Zi*)
    d. Herba Artemisiae Capillaris (*Yin Chen Hao*)
    e. Fructus Amomi Tsao-kuo (*Cao Guo*)

    Answer: ___

142. The modern standard dosage range for Semen Phaseoli Calcarati (*Chi Xiao Dou*) runs from:
   a. 3-9g
   b. 4.5-12g
   c. 9-30g
   d. 12-15g
   e. 1.5-3g

   Answer: ___

143. What medicinal is often combined with kidney yang supplements in order to prevent upward stirring of ministerial fire:
   a. Rhizoma Alismatis (*Ze Xie*)
   b. Bulbus Fritillariae Cirrhosae (*Chuan Bei Me*)
   c. Rhizoma Coptidis Chinensis (*Huang Lian*)
   d. Rhizoma Cyperi Rotundi (*Xiang Fu*)
   e. Radix Bupleuri (*Chai Hu*)

   Answer: ___

144. Both Caulis Akebiae (*Mu Tong*) and Medulla Tetrapanacis Papyriferi (*Tong Cao*) clear heat and eliminate dampness. However, which one is better for clearing heat:
   a. Medulla Tetrapanacis Papyriferi (*Tong Cao*)
   b. Caulis Akebiae (*Mu Tong*)

   Answer: ___

145. Which of the following medicinals A) disinhibits urination and frees the flow of strangury and B) frees the flow of the breast milk:
   a. Semen Plantaginis (*Che Qian Zi*)
   b. Talcum (*Hua Shi*)
   c. Squama Manitis Pentadactylis (*Chuan Shan Jia*)
   d. Caulis Akebiae (*Mu Tong*)
   e. Rhizoma Alismatis (*Ze Xie*)

   Answer: ___

146. Which of the following medicinals is best for red urination, vexation and agitation, and sores in the mouth and on the tongue:
   a. Sclerotium Poriae Cocos (*Fu Ling*)
   b. Sclerotium Polypori Umbellati (*Zhu Ling*)
   c. Caulis Akebiae (*Mu Tong*)
   d. Talcum (*Hua Shi*)
   e. Semen Abutilonis Seu Malvae (*Dong Kui Zi*)

   Answer: ___

147. Which of the following is not a function of Semen Plantaginis (*Che Qian Zi*):
    a. Clears the lungs and transforms phlegm
    b. Clears the liver and brightens the eyes
    c. Disinhibits urination and frees the flow of strangury
    d. Seeps dampness and stops diarrhea
    e. Clears heat and resolves toxins

    Answer: ___

148. Semen Plantaginis (*Che Qian Zi*) should be:
    a. Wrapped for decoction
    b. Decocted first
    c. Decocted later
    d. Steeped
    e. Smashed

    Answer: ___

149. Which of the following medicinals is best for treating damp heat strangury:
    a. Sclerotium Poriae Cocos (*Fu Ling*)
    b. Sclerotium Polypori Umbellati (*Zhu Ling*)
    c. Rhizoma Alismatis (*Ze Xie*)
    d. Talcum (*Hua Shi*)
    e. Gypsum Fibrosum (*Shi Gao*)

    Answer: ___

150. Which of the following medicinals should be wrapped during decoction:
    a. Talcum (*Hua Shi*)
    b. Gypsum Fibrosum (*Shi Gao*)
    c. Concha Ostreae (*Mu Li*)
    d. Dens Draconis (*Long Chi*)
    e. Carapax Amydae Sinensis (*Bei Jia*)

    Answer: ___

151. Which medicinal treats both painful urination and constipation with dry stools:
    a. Herba Dianthi (*Qu Mai*)
    b. Medulla Junci Effusi (*Deng Xin Cao*)
    c. Medulla Tetrapanacis Papyriferi (*Tong Cao*)
    d. Semen Abutilonis Seu Malvae (*Dong Kui Zi*)
    e. Herba Polygoni Avicularis (*Bian Xu*)

    Answer: ___

152. Which is the best of the following medicinals for treating damp heat skin diseases:
    a. Fructus Kochiae Scopariae (*Di Fu Zi*)
    b. Cortex Benincasae Hispidae (*Dong Gua Pi*)
    c. Semen Phaseoli Calcarati (*Chi Xiao Dou*)
    d. Herba Equiseti Hiemalis (*Mu Zei Cao*)
    e. Herba Polygoni Avicularis (*Bian Xu*)

    Answer: ___

153. Herba Desmodii Styrachifolii (*Jin Qian Cao*) is best for treating:
    a. Heat & stone strangury
    b. Heat & blood strangury
    c. Stone & blood strangury
    d. Heat & turbid strangury
    e. All of the above

    Answer: ___

154. Which of the following medicinals is best for treating damp heat jaundice:
    a. Herba Desmodii Styrachifolii (*Jin Qian Cao*)
    b. Herba Artemisae Capillaris (*Yin Chen Hao*)
    c. Spora Lygodii Japonici (*Hai Jin Sha*)
    d. Herba Pyrossiae (*Shi Wei*)
    e. Herba Andrographidis Paniculatae (*Chuan Xin Lian*)

    Answer: ___

155. Medulla Junci Effusi (*Deng Xin Cao*)'s functions are to:
    a. Disinhibit urination, seep dampness, and dispel wind heat
    b. Disinhibit urination, free the flow of strangury, clear heat, and eliminate vexation
    c. Clear heat, eliminate vexation, out-thrust rashes, and stop itching
    d. Disinhibit urination, disperse swelling, and quiet the spirit
    e. Clear heat, stop vomiting, eliminate vexation, and stop thirst

    Answer: ___

156. Herba Polygoni Avicularis (*Bian Xu*)'s functions are to:
    a. Disinhibit urination, disperse swelling, stop cough, and transform phlegm
    b. Disinhibit urination, disperse swelling, resolve toxins, and discharge pus
    c. Disinhibit urination, disperse swelling, clear heat, and free the flow of strangury
    d. Disinhibit urination, free the flow of strangury, kills worms, and stop itching
    e. Disinhibit urination, free the flow of strangury, and divide clear from turbid

    Answer: ___

157. Both Sclerotium Poriae Cocos (*Fu Ling*) and Semen Coicis Lachryma-jobi (*Yi Yi Ren*):
    a. Disinhibit urination, seep dampness, and recede or abate jaundice
    b. Disinhibit urination, seep dampness, and discharge pus
    c. Disinhibit urination, seep dampness, and quiet the spirit
    d. Disinhibit urination, seep dampness, and fortify the spleen
    e. Disinhibit urination, seep dampness, and free the flow of breast milk

    Answer: ___

158. Both Caulis Akebiae (*Mu Tong*) and Medulla Tetrapanacis Papyriferi (*Tong Cao*):
    a. Disinhibit urination, free the flow of strangury, dispel wind and free the flow of the network vessels
    b. Disinhibit urination, free the flow of strangury, and stop lactation
    c. Disinhibit urination, clear heat, and free the flow of breast milk
    d. Disinhibit urination, free the flow of strangury, quicken the blood and free the flow of the network vessels
    e. None of the above

    Answer: ___

Wind Dampness Treating Medicinals (*Zhi Feng Shi Yao*)

159. Which medicinal A) dispels wind dampness and B) resolves the exterior:
    a. Radix Gentianae Macrophyllae (*Qin Jiao*)
    b. Ramulus Mori Albi (*Sang Zhi*)
    c. Radix Stephaniae Tetrandrae (*Han Fang Ji*)
    d. Radix Angelicae Pubescentis (*Du Huo*)
    e. Radix Clematidis Chinensis (*Wei Ling Xian*)

    Answer: ___

160. Radix Angelicae Pubescentis (*Du Huo*) gathers in or enters which "channels":
    a. Kidney & heart
    b. Kidney & bladder
    c. Kidney & liver
    d. Liver and bladder
    e. Bladder and gallbladder

    Answer: ___

161. Which wind damp medicinal A) dispels wind dampness, B) clears vacuity heat, and C) moistens the intestines:
    a. Semen Pruni Persicae (*Tao Ren*)
    b. Semen Cannabis Sativae (*Huo Ma Ren*)
    c. Radix Angelicae Pubescentis (*Du Huo*)
    d. Radix Gentianae Macrophyllae (*Qin Jiao*)
    e. Radix Ledebouriellae Divaricatae (*Fang Feng*)

    Answer: ___

162. Radix Clematidis Chinensis (*Wei Ling Xian*) should be combined with _____ for wind damp impediment pain in the lower extremities:
    a. Radix Et Rhizoma Notoptergyii (*Qiang Huo*)
    b. Radix Ledebouriellae Divaricatae (*Fang Feng*)
    c. Radix Angelicae Pubescentis (*Du Huo*)
    d. cooked Radix Rehmanniae (*Shu Di*)
    e. Radix Achyranthis Bidentatae (*Niu Xi*)

    Answer: ___

163. A good medicinal for wind damp cold impediment pain complicated by liver-kidney vacuity is:
    a. Radix Et Rhizoma Notoptergyii (*Qiang Huo*)
    b. Radix Ledebouriellae Divaricatae (*Fang Feng*)
    c. Radix Angelicae Pubescentis (*Du Huo*)
    d. cooked Radix Rehmanniae (*Shu Di*)
    e. Cortex Radicis Acanthopanacis Gracilistyli (*Wu Jia Pi*)

    Answer: ___

164. Which of the following medicinals is good for damp heat impediment with red, swollen joints:
    a. Radix Ledebouriellae Divaricatae (*Fang Feng*)
    b. Herba Asari Cum Radice (*Xi Xin*)
    c. Radix Gentianae Macrophyllae (*Qin Jiao*)
    d. Radix Angelicae Pubescentis (*Du Huo*)
    e. Radix Clematidis Chinensis (*Wei Ling Xian*)

    Answer: ___

165. Which medicinal mainly treats upper extremity impediment pain:
    a. Folium Mori Albi (*Sang Ye*)
    b. Cortex Radicis Mori Albi (*Sang Bai Pi*)
    c. Ramulus Loranthi Seu Visci (*Sang Ji Sheng*)
    d. Fructus Mori Albi (*Sang Shen*)
    e. Ramulus Mori Albi (*Sang Zhi*)

    Answer: ___

166. Which of the following medicinals dispels wind, frees the flow of the network vessels, and settles fright:
    a. Agkistrodon Seu Bungarus (*Bai Hua She*)
    b. Herba Asari Cum Radice (*Xi Xin*)
    c. Ramulus Mori Albi (*Sang Zhi*)
    d. Caulis Trachelospermi Jasminoidis (*Luo Shi Teng*)
    e. Fructus Chaenomelis Lagenariae (*Mu Gua*)

    Answer: ___

167. Which of the following medicinals treats both vomiting and diarrhea and muscle spasms:
    a. Rhizoma Coptidis Chinensis (*Huang Lian*)
    b. Fructus Evodiae Rutecarpae (*Wu Zhu Yu*)
    c. Fructus Chaenomelis Lagenariae (*Mu Gua*)
    d. Semen Coicis Lachryma-jobi (*Yi Yi Ren*)
    e. Rhizoma Pinelliae Ternatae (*Ban Xia*)

    Answer: ___

168. Radix Stephaniae Tetrandrae (*Han Fang Ji*) is best for treating:
    a. Cold damp impediment
    b. Damp heat impediment
    c. Kidney vacuity low back pain
    d. Vomiting and diarrhea with muscle spasms
    e. Fishbone stuck in the throat

    Answer: ___

169. Which of the following medicinals A) dispels wind damp and B) supplements the liver and kidneys:
    a. Ramulus Loranthi Seu Visci (*Sang Ji Sheng*)
    b. Cortex Eucommiae Ulmoidis (*Du Zhong*)
    c. Radix Achyranthis Bidentatae (*Niu Xi*)
    d. Radix Dipsaci (*Xu Duan*)
    e. Fructus Psoraleae Corylifoliae (*Bu Gu Zhi*)

    Answer: ___

170. All of the following medicinals dispel wind dampness and are cool or cold in nature except:
    a. Radix Stephaniae Tetrandrae (*Han Fang Ji*)
    b. Radix Gentianae Macrophyllae (*Qin Jiao*)
    c. Herba Siegesbeckiae (*Xi Xian Cao*)
    d. Caulis Trachelospermi Jasminoidis (*Luo Shi Teng*)
    e. Herba Asari Cum Radice (*Xi Xin*)

    Answer: ___

Phlegm-transforming, Cough-stopping Medicinals (*Hua Tan Zhi Ke Yao*)

171. Which medicinal is not cool or cold and, therefore, is not usually used to treat phlegm heat:
    a. Radix Peucedani (*Qian Hu*)
    b. Bulbus Fritillariae Thunbergii (*Zhe Bei Mu*)
    c. Semen Sinapis Albae (*Bai Jie Zi*)
    d. Fructus Trichosanthis Kirlowii (*Gua Lou*)
    e. Caulis Bambusae In Taeniis (*Zhu Ru*)

    Answer: ___

172. Which part of Trichosanthes is best to use if there is phlegm heat with lung-stomach fluid dryness:
    a. Semen Trichosanthis Kirlowii (*Gua Lou Ren*)
    b. Pericarpium Trichosanthis Kirlowii (*Gua Lou Pi*)
    c. whole Fructus Trichosanthis Kirlowii (*Quan Gua Lou*)
    d. Radix Trichosanthis Kirlowii (*Tian Hua Fen*)

    Answer: ___

173. The qi of Radix Platycodi Grandiflori (*Jie Geng*) is:
    a. Upbearing
    b. Downbearing
    c. Entering
    d. Out-thrusting

    Answer: ___

174. Chinese medical theory posits a correspondence between the lungs and the skin. What medicinal which stops coughing and levels panting treats coughing when taken internally and various skin conditions when applied externally:
    a. Fructus Perillae Frutescentis (*Zi Su Zi*)
    b. Herba Ephedrae (*Ma Huang*)
    c. Radix Stemonae (*Bai Bu*)
    d. Radix Platycodi Grandiflori (*Jie Geng*)
    e. Radix Peucedani (*Qian Hu*)

    Answer: ___

175. Rhizoma Pinelliae Ternatae (*Ban Xia*)'s functions are to:
    a. Dry dampness and transform phlegm, downbear counterflow and stop vomiting
    b. Clear heat and transform phlegm, downbear counterflow and stop vomiting
    c. Warmly transform cold phlegm, warm the middle, and stop diarrhea
    d. Warm the lungs and transform phlegm, kill worms and stop diarrhea
    e. Warm the lungs and transform phlegm, disinhibit urination and disperse swelling

    Answer: ___

176. The qi of Cortex Magnoliae Officinalis (*Hou Po*) is:
    a. Upbearing
    b. Downbearing
    c. Entering
    d. Out-thrusting

    Answer: ___

177. Rhizoma Pinelliae Ternatae (*Ban Xia*) is commonly combined with which of the following medicinals in order to treat dampness and phlegm:
    a. Rhizoma Atractylodis (*Cang Zhu*) & Semen Coicis Lachryma-jobi (*Yi Yi Ren*)
    b. Cortex Magnoliae Officinalis (*Hou Po*) & Semen Dolichoris Lablab (*Bai Bian Dou*)
    c. Pericarpium Citri Reticulatae (*Chen Pi*) & Sclerotium Poriae Cocos (*Fu Ling*)
    d. Rhizoma Atractylodis Macrocephalae (*Bai Zhu*) & Fructus Cardamomi (*Bai Dou Kou*)
    e. Fructus Amomi (*Sha Ren*) & Fructus Citri Sacrodactylis (*Fo Shou*)

    Answer: ___

178. Which of the following medicinals is the best one to treat chest impediment:
    a. whole Fructus Trichosanthis Kirlowii (*Quan Gua Lou*)
    b. Bulbus Fritillariae Thunbergii (*Zhe Bei Mu*)
    c. Rhizoma Arisaematis (*Nan Xing*)
    d. Radix Platycodi Grandiflori (*Jie Geng*)
    e. Pericarpium Citri Reticulatae (*Chen Pi*)

    Answer: ___

179. Radix Coreani Seu Typhonii (*Bai Fu Zi*)'s functions are to:
    a. Dry dampness and transform phlegm, dispel wind and stop tetany
    b. Dry dampness and transform phlegm, harmonize the stomach and stop vomiting
    c. Dry dampness and transform phlegm, warm the lungs and stop coughing
    d. Dry dampness and transform phlegm, dispel wind and scatter cold
    e. Dry dampness and transform phlegm, boost the qi and open the orifices

    Answer: ___

180. Which of the following medicinals is best for the treatment of wind phlegm with heat:
    a. Bombyx Batryticatus (*Jiang Can*)
    b. Radix Coreani Seu Typhonii (*Bai Fu Zi*)
    c. bile-treated Rhizoma Arisaematis (*Dan Nan Xing*)
    d. Fructus Gleditschiae Chinensis (*Zao Jiao*)
    e. Rhizoma Arisaematis (*Tian Nan Xing*)

    Answer: ___

181. Which of the following medicinals is best for the treatment of cough with profuse phlegm, chest oppression, and sore throat or loss of voice:
    a. Fructus Arctii Lappae (*Niu Bang Zi*)
    b. Pericarpium Citri Reticulatae (*Chen Pi*)
    c. Rhizoma Pinelliae Ternatae (*Ban Xia*)
    d. Semen Sinapis Albae (*Bai Jie Zi*)
    e. Radix Platycodi Grandiflori (*Jie Geng*)

    Answer: ___

182. Which medicinal upbears the qi, diffuses the lungs, and expels phlegm:
    a. Flos Inulae (*Xuan Fu Hua*)
    b. Radix Platycodi Grandiflori (*Jie Geng*)
    c. Semen Pruni Armeniacae (*Xing Ren*)
    d. Radix Peucedani (*Qian Hu*)
    e. Fructus Perillae Frutescentis (*Zi Su Zi*)

    Answer: ___

183. Which of the following medicinals A) clears lung and stomach heat and transforms phlegm and B) rectifies the qi and loosens the chest:
    a. Semen Pruni Armeniacae (*Xing Ren*)
    b. Folium Eriobotryae Japonicae (*Pi Pa Ye*)
    c. Cortex Radicis Mori Albi (*Sang Bai Pi*)
    d. Fructus Trichosanthis Kirlowii (*Gua Lou*)
    e. Radix Stemonae (*Bai Bu*)

    Answer: ___

184. Which of the following medicinals A) clears the lungs and transforms phlegm and B) moistens the intestines and frees the flow of the stool:
    a. Semen Trichosanthis Kirlowii (*Gua Lou Ren*)
    b. Semen Pruni Armeniacae (*Xing Ren*)
    c. Fructus Perillae Frutescentis (*Zi Su Zi*)
    d. Caulis Bambusae In Taeniis (*Zhu Ru*)
    e. Bulbus Fritillariae Thunbergii (*Zhe Bei Mu*)

    Answer: ___

185. Which of the following medicinals is most effective for draining the lungs and leveling panting:
    a. Fructus Perillae Frutescentis (*Zi Su Zi*)
    b. Cortex Radicis Mori Albi (*Sang Bai Pi*)
    c. Radix Platycodi Grandiflori (*Jie Geng*)
    d. Radix Scutellariae Baicalensis (*Huang Qin*)
    e. Semen Ginkgonis Bilobae (*Bai Guo*)

    Answer: ___

186. The common functions of Thallus Algae (*Kun Bu*) and Herba Sargassii (*Hai Zao*) are to:
    a. Warm the lungs and expel phlegm
    b. Dry dampness and transform phlegm
    c. Soften the hard and transform phlegm
    d. Soften the hard and precipitate downward
    e. All of the above

    Answer: ___

187. Which of the following medicinals is the best for treating pain and numbness in the extremities and joints:
    a. Fructus Gleditschiae Chinensis (*Zao Jiao*)
    b. Bulbus Fritillariae Thunbergii (*Zhe Bei Mu*)
    c. Flos Inulae (*Xuan Fu Hua*)
    d. Semen Sinapis Albae (*Bai Jie Zi*)
    e. Rhizoma Pinelliae Ternatae (*Ban Xia*)

    Answer: ___

188. The flavor and nature (*i.e.*, temperature) of Bulbus Fritillariae Thunbergii (*Zhe Bei Mu*) are:
    a. Bitter & cold
    b. Sweet & cold
    c. Salty & cold
    d. Bitter & warm
    e. None of the above

    Answer: ___

189. Which medicinal A) stops cough and levels panting and B) moistens the intestines and frees the flow of the stool:
    a. Semen Trichosanthis Kirlowii (*Gua Lou Ren*)
    b. Semen Tinglizi (*Ting Li Zi*)
    c. Semen Cannabis Sativae (*Huo Ma Ren*)
    d. Semen Pruni Armeniacae (*Xing Ren*)
    e. Semen Sinapis Albae (*Bai Jie Zi*)

    Answer: ___

190. Fructus Perillae Frutescentis (*Zi Su Zi*)'s functions are to:
    a. Clear the lungs and transform phlegm
    b. Moisten the lungs and transform phlegm
    c. Downbear counterflow and transform phlegm
    d. Dry dampness and transform phlegm
    e. Clear heat and moisten the intestines

    Answer: ___

191. Which of the following medicinals is commonly used in repletion patterns of edema and ascites:
    a. Flos Inulae (*Xuan Fu Hua*)
    b. Semen Tinglizi (*Ting Li Zi*)
    c. Cortex Radicis Mori Albi (*Sang Bai Pi*)
    d. Radix Stemonae (*Bai Bu*)
    e. Semen Raphani Sativi (*Lai Fu Zi*)

    Answer: ___

192. Folium Eriobotryae Japonicae (*Pi Pa Ye*) not only transforms phlegm and stops cough but also:
    a. Disinhibits urination and disperses swelling
    b. Dispels wind and clears heat
    c. Harmonizes the stomach and downbears counterflow
    d. Nourishes the liver and extinguishes wind
    e. Relaxes tension (spasm and contractions) and soothes the sinews

    Answer: ___

193. Which medicinal secures the lungs and levels panting at the same time as eliminating dampness and stopping abnormal vaginal discharge:
    a. Semen Pruni Armeniacae (*Xing Ren*)
    b. Radix Angelicae Dahuricae (*Bai Zhi*)
    c. Semen Ginkgonis Bilobae (*Bai Guo*)
    d. Semen Euryalis Ferocis (*Qian Shi*)
    e. Radix Platycodi Grandiflori (*Jie Geng*)

    Answer: ___

194. Semen Sinapis Albae (*Bai Jie Zi*), Fructus Perillae Frutescentis (*Zi Su Zi*), and Radix Coreani Seu Typhonii (*Bai Fu Zi*) all:
    a. Transform phlegm
    b. Level panting
    c. Stop coughing
    d. Dispel wind
    e. Moisten the intestines

    Answer: ___

195. Both Caulis Bambusae In Taeniis (*Zhu Ru*) and Folium Eriobotryae Japonicae (*Pi Pa Ye*):
    a. Clear heat and eliminate vexation
    b. Harmonize the stomach and downbear counterflow
    c. Secure the lungs and stop cough
    d. Clear heat and extinguish wind
    e. None of the above

    Answer: ___

196. Both Radix Asteris Tatarici (*Zi Wan*) and Flos Tussilaginis Farfarae (*Kuan Dong Hua*):
    a. Clear the lungs, stop coughing, and transform phlegm
    b. Drain the lungs, stop coughing, and level panting
    c. Moisten the lungs, stop coughing, and transform phlegm
    d. Secure the lungs, stop coughing, and level panting
    e. None of the above

    Answer: ___

197. Which medicinals transform phlegm and scatter nodulation:
    a. Radix Platycodi Grandiflori (*Jie Geng*) & Caulis Bambusae In Taeniis (*Zhu Ru*)
    b. Semen Pruni Armeniacae (*Xing Ren*) & Radix Peucedani (*Qian Hu*)
    c. Herba Sargassii (*Hai Zao*) & Concha Cyclinae Sinensis (*Hai Ge Ke*)
    d. Folium Eriobotryae Japonicae (*Pi Pa Ye*) & Semen Ginkgonis Bilobae (*Bai Guo*)
    e. Radix Stemonae (*Bai Bu*) & Fructus Perillae Frutescentis (*Zi Su Zi*)

    Answer: ___

198. Which medicinals are A) warm but not dry, B) moistening but not slimy, and C) stop cough and level panting:
    a. Semen Pruni Armeniacae (*Xing Ren*) & Semen Ginkgonis Bilobae (*Bai Guo*)
    b. Cortex Radicis Mori Albi (*Sang Bai Pi*) & Semen Tinglizi (*Ting Li Zi*)
    c. Fructus Perillae Frutescentis (*Zi Su Zi*) & Folium Eriobotryae Japonicae (*Pi Pa Ye*)
    d. Radix Stemonae (*Bai Bu*) & Radix Asteris Tatarici (*Zi Wan*)
    e. Herba Houttuyniae Cordatae Cum Radice (*Yu Xing Cao*) & Tuber Ophiopogonis Japonici (*Mai Men Dong*)

    Answer: ___

199. Which of the following medicinals moistens the lungs and stops cough as well as kills worms:
    a. Radix Asteris Tatarici (*Zi Wan*)
    b. Radix Stemonae (*Bai Bu*)
    c. Flos Tussilaginis Farfarae (*Kuan Dong Hua*)
    d. Bulbus Fritillariae Cirrhosae (*Chuan Bei Mu*)
    e. Semen Pruni Armeniacae (*Xing Ren*)

    Answer: ___

200. Which of the following medicinals treats hoarse voice:
    a. Rhizoma Pinelliae Ternatae (*Ban Xia*)
    b. Radix Platycodi Grandiflori (*Jie Geng*)
    c. Caulis Bambusae In Taeniis (*Zhu Ru*)
    d. Rhizoma Arisaematis (*Nan Xing*)
    e. Bulbus Fritillariae Thunbergii (*Zhe Bei Mu*)

    Answer: ___

201. Both Rhizoma Pinelliae Ternatae (*Ban Xia*) and Caulis Bambusae In Taeniis (*Zhu Ru*):
   a. Transform phlegm and soothe the liver
   b. Transform phlegm and rectify the qi
   c. Transform phlegm and disinhibit urination
   d. Transform phlegm and stop vomiting
   e. Transform phlegm and settle fright

   Answer: ___

Food-dispersing Medicinals (*Xiao Shi Yao*)

202. Which medicinal is best for meaty type food stagnation:
    a. Semen Raphani Sativi (*Lai Fu Zi*)
    b. Fructus Germinatus Hordei Vulgaris (*Mai Ya*)
    c. Fructus Germinatus Oryzae Sativae (*Gu Ya*)
    d. Massa Medica Fermentata (*Shen Qu*)
    e. Fructus Crataegi (*Shan Zha*)

    Answer: ___

203. Large doses of stir-fried Fructus Germinatus Hordei Vulgaris (*Mai Ya*) can:
    a. Hasten birth
    b. Quiet the fetus
    c. Secure desertion
    d. Stop bleeding
    e. Stop lactation

    Answer: ___

204. Endothelium Corneum Gigeriae Galli (*Ji Nei Jin*) is often combined with Herba Lysimachiae (*Jin Qian Cao*) for the treatment of:
    a. Seminal emission
    b. Constipation
    c. Early menstruation
    d. Urinary and/or biliary tract stones
    e. This is an impossible combination

    Answer: ___

205. Which of the following medicinals quickens the blood and dispels stasis:
    a. Massa Medica Fermentata (*Shen Qu*)
    b. Endothelium Corneum Gigeriae Galli (*Ji Nei Jin*)
    c. Fructus Germinatus Hordei Vulgaris (*Mai Ya*)
    d. Fructus Germinatus Oryzae Sativae (*Gu Ya*)
    e. Fructus Crataegi (*Shan Zha*)

    Answer: ___

206. The main functions of Semen Raphani Sativi (*Lai Fu Zi*) are to:
    a. Disperse food and abduct stagnation, fortify the spleen and harmonize the middle
    b. Disperse food and abduct stagnation, fortify the spleen and boost the stomach
    c. Disperse food and abduct stagnation, rectify the qi and resolve depression
    d. Disperse food and abduct stagnation, supplement the kidneys and warm yang
    e. Disperse food and abduct stagnation, downbear the qi and transform phlegm

    Answer: ___

207. The main functions of Endothelium Corneum Gigeriae Galli (*Ji Nei Jin*) are to:
   a. Disperse food and abduct stagnation, disinhibit urination and break stones
   b. Disperse food and abduct stagnation, fortify the spleen and clear and eliminate dampness and heat
   c. Disperse food and abduct stagnation, enrich yin and clear vacuity heat
   d. Disperse food and abduct stagnation, supplement the kidneys and warm yang
   e. Disperse food and abduct stagnation, nourish the liver and boost the essence

   Answer: ___

208. Which of the following medicinals is commonly taken as a powder or pill:
   a. Massa Medica Fermentata (*Shen Qu*)
   b. Semen Raphani Sativi (*Lai Fu Zi*)
   c. Endothelium Corneum Gigeriae Galli (*Ji Nei Jin*)
   d. Fructus Germinatus Hordei Vulgaris (*Mai Ya*)
   e. Fructus Germinatus Oryzae Sativae (*Gu Ya*)

   Answer: ___

Qi-rectifying Medicinals (*Li Qi Yao*)

209. Pericarpium Citri Reticulatae (*Chen Pi*) gathers in or enters which "channels":
   a. Lung, spleen, and large intestine
   b. Lung, spleen, and stomach
   c. Lung, heart, and liver
   d. Lung, liver, and large intestine
   e. Stomach, large intestine, and bladder

   Answer: ___

210. Which moves the qi more forcefully:
   a. Pericarpium Citri Reticulatae Viride (*Qing Pi*)
   b. Pericarpium Citri Reticulatae (*Chen Pi*)

   Answer: ___

211. Which moves the qi more forcefully:
   a. Fructus Citri Aurantii (*Zhi Ke*)
   b. Fructus Immaturus Citri Aurantii (*Zhi Shi*)

   Answer: ___

212. Which qi-rectifying medicinal also fortifies the spleen:
   a. Rhizoma Cyperi Rotundi (*Xiang Fu*)
   b. Radix Bupleuri (*Chai Hu*)
   c. Radix Auklandiae Lappae (*Mu Xiang*)
   d. Fructus Citri Aurantii (*Zhi Ke*)
   e. Fructus Meliae Toosendan (*Chuan Lian Zi*)

   Answer: ___

213. Which qi-rectifying medicinal not only moves the qi and stops pain but warms the kidneys:
   a. Rhizoma Cyperi Rotundi (*Xiang Fu*)
   b. Radix Bupleuri (*Chai Hu*)
   c. Radix Auklandiae Lappae (*Mu Xiang*)
   d. Fructus Meliae Toosendan (*Chuan Lian Zi*)
   e. Radix Linderae Strychnifoliae (*Wu Yao*)

   Answer: ___

214. Which qi-rectifying medicinal A) clears heat and eliminates dampness and B) kills parasites:
   a. Rhizoma Cyperi Rotundi (*Xiang Fu*)
   b. Radix Bupleuri (*Chai Hu*)
   c. Radix Auklandiae Lappae (*Mu Xiang*)
   d. Fructus Meliae Toosendan (*Chuan Lian Zi*)
   e. Radix Linderae Strychnifoliae (*Wu Yao*)

   Answer: ___

215. Which is not a function of Pericarpium Citri Reticulatae (*Chen Pi*):
    a. Dries dampness and transforms phlegm
    b. Downbears counterflow
    c. Fortifies the spleen
    d. Disperses stagnation
    e. Harmonizes the middle

    Answer: ___

216. Which of the following medicinals is the best for spleen-stomach qi stagnation with abdominal distention, belching, nausea, and vomiting:
    a. Pericarpium Citri Reticulatae (*Chen Pi*)
    b. Rhizoma Pinelliae Ternatae (*Ban Xia*)
    c. Sclerotium Poriae Cocos (*Fu Ling*)
    d. Cortex Magnoliae Officinalis (*Hou Po*)
    e. Rhizoma Atractylodis (*Cang Zhu*)

    Answer: ___

217. Which of the following medicinals gathers in or enters the lung channel:
    a. Pericarpium Citri Reticulatae Viride (*Qing Pi*)
    b. Fructus Citri Aurantii (*Zhi Ke*)
    c. Pericarpium Citri Reticulatae (*Chen Pi*)
    d. Fructus Citri Sacrodactylis (*Fo Shou*)
    e. Radix Auklandiae Lappae (*Mu Xiang*)

    Answer: ___

218. Which of the following medicinals can break the qi and transform phlegm:
    a. Pericarpium Citri Reticulatae (*Chen Pi*)
    b. Rhizoma Pinelliae Ternatae (*Ban Xia*)
    c. Cortex Magnoliae Officinalis (*Hou Po*)
    d. Fructus Immaturus Citri Aurantii (*Zhi Shi*)
    e. Fructus Citri Sacrodactylis (*Fo Shou*)

    Answer: ___

219. Which of the following medicinals is bitter, acrid, and slightly cold or cool:
    a. Pericarpium Citri Reticulatae (*Chen Pi*)
    b. Pericarpium Citri Reticulatae Viride (*Qing Pi*)
    c. Fructus Immaturus Citri Aurantii (*Zhi Shi*)
    d. Fructus Citri Sacrodactylis (*Fo Shou*)
    e. Fructus Amomi (*Sha Ren*)

    Answer: ___

220. Which of the following medicinals rectifies the qi and stops pain and is effective for treating spleen-stomach qi stagnation:
    a. Radix Auklandiae Lappae (*Mu Xiang*)
    b. Rhizoma Cyperi Rotundi (*Xiang Fu*)
    c. Fructus Meliae Toosendan (*Chuan Lian Zi*)
    d. Semen Litchi Chinensis (*Li Zhi He*)
    e. Radix Linderae Strychnifoliae (*Wu Yao*)

    Answer: ___

221. What are the functions of Radix Linderae Strychnifoliae (*Wu Yao*):
    a. Rectifies the qi, harmonizes the middle, and stops pain
    b. Downbears counterflow, harmonizes the middle, and stops pain
    c. Rectifies the qi and stops pain, scatters cold and disperses stagnation
    d. Frees the flow of yang and disperses stagnation
    e. Rectifies the qi and stops pain, warms the kidneys and scatters cold

    Answer: ___

222. Which of the following medicinals A) rectifies the qi and stops pain and B) warms the kidneys and promotes their absorption or grasping of the qi:
    a. Magnetitum (*Ci Shi*)
    b. Lignum Aquilariae Agallochae (*Chen Xiang*)
    c. Fructus Psoraleae Corylifoliae (*Bu Gu Zhi*)
    d. Radix Linderae Strychnifoliae (*Wu Yao*)
    e. Gecko (*Ge Jie*)

    Answer: ___

223. Which of the following medicinals is best for treating kidney yang vacuity frequent urination:
    a. Fructus Zanthoxyli Bungeani (*Hua Jiao*)
    b. Fructus Evodiae Rutecarpae (*Wu Zhu Yu*)
    c. Radix Auklandiae Lappae (*Mu Xiang*)
    d. Radix Linderae Strychnifoliae (*Wu Yao*)
    e. dry Rhizoma Zingiberis (*Gan Jiang*)

    Answer: ___

224. Which of the following medicinals is best for treating liver-stomach disharmony with rib-side pain, chest oppression, belching, nausea, and vomiting:
    a. Pericarpium Citri Reticulatae (*Chen Pi*)
    b. Fructus Citri Aurantii (*Zhi Ke*)
    c. Radix Linderae Strychnifoliae (*Wu Yao*)
    d. Fructus Citri Sacrodactylis (*Fo Shou*)
    e. Lignum Aquilariae Agallochae (*Chen Xiang*)

    Answer: ___

225. Rhizoma Cyperi Rotundi (*Xiang Fu*)'s functions are to:
    a. Emolliate the liver
    b. Course the liver
    c. Subdue the liver
    d. Clear the liver
    e. Nourish the liver

    Answer: ___

226. Which of the following medicinals A) courses the liver and rectifies the qi and B) regulates menstruation and stops pain:
    a. Radix Angelicae Sinensis (*Dang Gui*)
    b. Rhizoma Cyperi Rotundi (*Xiang Fu*)
    c. Fructus Meliae Toosendan (*Chuan Lian Zi*)
    d. Radix Albus Paeoniae Lactiflorae (*Bai Shao*)
    e. Lignum Aquilariae Agallochae (*Chen Xiang*)

    Answer: ___

227. Which of the following medicinals is best for heat pattern qi mounting lower abdominal and testicular pain:
    a. Semen Litchi Chinensis (*Li Zhi He*)
    b. Fructus Foeniculi Vulgaris (*Xiao Hui Xiang*)
    c. Radix Linderae Strychnifoliae (*Wu Yao*)
    d. Pericarpium Citri Reticulatae (*Chen Pi*)
    e. Fructus Meliae Toosendan (*Chuan Lian Zi*)

    Answer: ___

228. Which of the following medicinals rectifies the qi and disperses stagnation, frees the flow of yang and loosens the chest in case of chest impediment:
    a. Bulbus Allii (*Xie Bai*)
    b. Ramulus Cinnamomi Cassiae (*Gui Zhi*)
    c. Fructus Trichosanthis Kirlowii (*Gua Lou*)
    d. Fructus Immaturus Citri Aurantii (*Zhi Shi*)
    e. Rhizoma Pinelliae Ternatae (*Ban Xia*)

    Answer: ___

Blood-rectifying Medicinals (*Li Xue Yao*)

229. There are four basic causes of pathological bleeding: 1) heat, 2) qi vacuity, 3) blood stasis, and 4) trauma severing the channels and vessels. Pollen Typhae (*Pu Huang*) is best for the treatment of bleeding due to which of these four:
    a. Heat
    b. Qi vacuity
    c. Blood stasis
    d. Trauma severing the channels and vessels
    e. A & B
    f. C & D

    Answer: ___

230. There are four basic causes of pathological bleeding: 1) heat, 2) qi vacuity, 3) blood stasis, and 4) trauma severing the channels and vessels. Herba Agrimoniae Pilosae (*Xian He Cao*) is best for the treatment of bleeding due to which of these four:
    a. Heat
    b. Qi vacuity
    c. Blood stasis
    d. Trauma severing the channels and vessels
    e. A & B
    f. C & D

    Answer: ___

231. There are four basic causes of pathological bleeding: 1) heat, 2) qi vacuity, 3) blood stasis, and 4) trauma severing the channels and vessels. Radix Sanguisorbae (*Di Yu*) is best for the treatment of bleeding due to which of these four:
    a. Heat
    b. Qi vacuity
    c. Blood stasis
    d. Trauma severing the channels and vessels
    e. A & B
    f. C & D

    Answer: ___

232. There are four basic causes of pathological bleeding: 1) heat, 2) qi vacuity, 3) blood stasis, and 4) trauma severing the channels and vessels. Radix Rubiae Cordifoliae (*Qian Cao Gen*) is best for the treatment of bleeding due to which of these four:
    a. Heat
    b. Qi vacuity
    c. Blood stasis
    d. Trauma severing the channels and vessels
    e. A & B
    f. C & D

    Answer: ___

233. Fructus Immaturus Sophorae Japonicae (*Huai Hua Mi*) is empirically especially famous for its
ability to treat _____ bleeding:
a. Oral
b. Ocular
c. Anal
d. Urinary
e. Aural

Answer: ___

234. Which of the following medicinals is best for treating hematuria:
a. Radix Sanguisorbae (*Di Yu*)
b. Cacumen Biotae Orientalis (*Ce Bai Ye*)
c. Herba Cephalanoploris Segeti (*Xiao Ji*)
d. Rhizoma Bletillae Striatae (*Bai Ji*)
e. Radix Rubiae Cordifoliae (*Qian Cao Gen*)

Answer: ___

235. Which of the following medicinals not only cools the blood and stops bleeding but also resolves
toxins and heals sores:
a. Radix Sanguisorbae (*Di Yu*)
b. Cacumen Biotae Orientalis (*Ce Bai Ye*)
c. Herba Cephalanoploris Segeti (*Xiao Ji*)
d. Rhizoma Bletillae Striatae (*Bai Ji*)
e. Radix Rubiae Cordifoliae (*Qian Cao Gen*)

Answer: ___

236. Which of the following pairs of medicinals treat blood heat hemafecia:
a. Crinis Carbonisatus (*Xue Yu Tan*) & Folium Artemisiae Argyii (*Ai Ye*)
b. carbonized Petiolus Trachycarpi (*Zong Lu Tan*) & Radix Pseudoginseng (*Tian San Qi*)
c. Radix Sanguisorbae (*Di Yu*) & Flos Immaturus Sophorae Japonicae (*Huai Hua Mi*)
d. Nodus Rhizomatis Nelumbinis Nuciferae (*Ou Jie*) & Terra Flava Ustae (*Fu Long Gan*)
e. Rhizoma Imperatae Cylindricae (*Bai Mao Gen*) & Os Sepiae Seu Sepiellae (*Wu Zei Gu*)

Answer: __

237. Rhizoma Imperatae Cylindricae (*Bai Mao Gen*)'s functions are to:
a. Cool the blood and stop bleeding, resolve toxins and heal sores
b. Cool the blood and stop bleeding, quicken the blood and dispel stasis
c. Cool the blood and stop bleeding, transform phlegm and stop coughing
d. Cool the blood and stop bleeding, clear heat and disinhibit urination
e. Cool the blood and stop bleeding, disperse food and abduct stagnation

Answer: ___

238. Cacumen Biotae Orientalis (*Ce Bai Ye*)'s functions are to:
    a. Cool the blood and stop bleeding, transform phlegm and stop cough
    b. Cool the blood and stop bleeding, quicken the blood and dispel stasis
    c. Cool the blood and stop bleeding, disperse swelling and welling abscesses
    d. Cool the blood and stop bleeding, resolve toxins and heal sores
    e. Cool the blood and stop bleeding, disperse swelling and engender new tissue

    Answer: ___

239. Herba Agrimoniae Pilosae (*Xian He Cao*)'s functions are to:
    a. Warm the channels & stop bleeding
    b. Astringe and secure & stop bleeding
    c. Dispel stasis & stop bleeding
    d. Cool the blood & stop bleeding
    e. Drain fire & stop bleeding

    Answer: ___

240. Rhizoma Bletillae Striatae (*Bai Ji*)'s functions are to:
    a. Astringe, secure, stop bleeding, dispel stasis and disperse swelling
    b. Astringe, secure, stop bleeding, disperse swelling and engender new tissue
    c. Astringe, secure, stop bleeding, resolve toxins and promote the closure (of sores)
    d. Cool the blood and stop bleeding, clear heat and resolve toxins
    e. Cool the blood and stop bleeding, transform phlegm and stop cough

    Answer: ___

241. Which of the following medicinals A) quickens the blood and stops pain and B) dispels stasis and stops bleeding:
    a. Resina Olibani (*Ru Xiang*)
    b. Radix Rubiae Cordifoliae (*Qian Cao Gen*)
    c. Rhizoma Corydalis Yanhusuo (*Yan Hu Suo*)
    d. Rhizoma Bletillae Striatae (*Bai Ji*)
    e. Radix Pseudoginseng (*Tian San Qi*)

    Answer: ___

242. Pollen Typhae (*Pu Huang*) should be:
    a. Decocted first
    b. Decocted later
    c. Dissolved in the strained decoction
    d. Wrapped during decoction
    e. Steeped

    Answer: ___

243. Which of the following medicinals is best for the treatment of vacuity cold uterine bleeding:
    a. Pollen Typhae (*Pu Huang*)
    b. Radix Sanguisorbae (*Di Yu*)
    c. Crinis Carbonisatus (*Xue Yu Tan*)
    d. Flos Immaturus Sophorae Japonicae (*Huai Hua Mi*)
    e. Folium Artemisiae Argyii (*Ai Ye*)

    Answer: ___

244. Which of the following medicinals is best for the treatment of vacuity cold uterine bleeding:
    a. blast-fried Rhizoma Zingiberis (*Pao Jiang*)
    b. Radix Rubiae Cordifoliae (*Qian Cao Gen*)
    c. Radix Scutellariae Baicalensis (*Huang Qin*)
    d. Nodus Rhizomatis Nelumbinis Nuciferae (*Ou Jie*)
    e. Rhizoma Guanchong (*Guan Zhong*)

    Answer: ___

245. Rhizoma Phragmitis Communis (*Lu Gen*) and Rhizoma Imperatae Cylindricae (*Bai Mao Gen*) both:
    a. Cool the blood and stop bleeding
    b. Drain fire and resolve toxins
    c. Clear heat and eliminate dampness
    d. Clear heat and disinhibit urination
    e. Disinhibit urination and disperse swelling

    Answer: ___

246. It is said that Radix Salviae Miltiorrhizae (*Dan Shen*) both nourishes and quickens the blood. However, which does it do more:
    a. Quickens
    b. Nourishes

    Answer: ___

247. Radix Ligustici Wallichii (*Chuan Xiong*) moves:
    a. The qi within the blood
    b. The blood within the blood
    c. The fluids within the blood
    d. The yin within the blood
    e. The defensive qi

    Answer: ___

248. Which of the following medicinals is best to treat impediment conditions and headache:
    a. Radix Auklandiae Lappae (*Mu Xiang*)
    b. Resina Olibani (*Ru Xiang*)
    c. Lignum Santali Albi (*Tan Xiang*)
    d. Rhizoma Cyperi Rotundi (*Xiang Fu*)
    e. Radix Ligustici Wallichii (*Chuan Xiong*)

    Answer: ___

249. Which medicinal A) dispels wind and stops pain and B) quickens the blood and rectifies the qi:
    a. Radix Salviae Miltiorrhizae (*Dan Shen*)
    b. Tuber Curcumae (*Yu Jin*)
    c. Resina Myrrhae (*Mo Yao*)
    d. Radix Ligustici Wallichii (*Chuan Xiong*)
    e. Flos Carthami Tinctorii (*Hong Hua*)

    Answer: ___

250. Which medicinal is said to "rise to the head and eyes and descend to the sea of blood":
    a. Flos Carthami Tinctorii (*Hong Hua*)
    b. Flos Chrysanthemi Morifolii (*Ju Hua*)
    c. Radix Ligustici Wallichii (*Chuan Xiong*)
    d. Radix Achyranthis Bidentatae (*Niu Xi*)
    e. Radix Bupleuri (*Chai Hu*)

    Answer: ___

251. Radix Ligustici Wallichii (*Chuan Xiong*)'s flavor and nature (*i.e.*, temperature) are:
    a. Sour & warm
    b. Bitter & cold
    c. Acrid & warm
    d. Acrid & cool
    e. Salty & level (*i.e.*, neutral)

    Answer: ___

252. There are two types of Peony (*Shao Yao*) — Radix Albus Paeoniae Lactiflorae (*Bai Shao*) and Radix Rubrus Paeoniae Lactiflorae (*Chi Shao*). One nourishes and restrains; the other cools and quickens. If one wants to cool the blood and/or quicken the blood, one should use:
    a. Radix Albus Paeoniae Lactiflorae (*Bai Shao*)
    b. Radix Rubrus Paeoniae Lactiflorae (*Chi Shao*)

    Answer: ___

253. Flos Carthami Tinctorii (*Hong Hua*) gathers in or enters which "channels":
    a. Liver & gallbladder
    b. Liver & stomach
    c. Liver & spleen
    d. Liver & large intestine
    e. Liver & heart

    Answer: ___

254. The duo, Rhizoma Sparganii (*San Leng*) and Rhizoma Curcumae Zedoariae (*E Zhu*):
    a. Quicken the blood and transform stasis
    b. Quicken the blood and dispel stasis
    c. Break the blood

    Answer: ___

255. The duo, Resina Olibani (*Ru Xiang*) and Resina Myrrhae (*Mo Yao*), are especially good for:
    a. Stopping vomiting
    b. Stopping diarrhea
    c. Stopping sweating
    d. Stopping pain
    e. Stopping cough

    Answer: ___

256. Which of the following pairs of medicinals quickens the blood and dispels stasis, disperses swelling and engenders new tissue:
    a. Resina Olibani (*Ru Xiang*) & Resina Myrrhae (*Mo Yao*)
    b. Rhizoma Sparganii (*San Leng*) & Rhizoma Curcumae Zedoariae (*E Zhu*)
    c. Radix Rubrus Paeoniae Lactiflorae (*Chi Shao*) & Cortex Radicis Moutan (*Dan Pi*)
    d. Radix Angelicae Dahuricae (*Bai Zhi*) & Radix Salviae Miltiorrhizae (*Dan Shen*)
    e. Pollen Typhae (*Pu Huang*) & Feces Trogopterori Seu Pteromi (*Wu Ling Zhi*)

    Answer: ___

257. Rhizoma Corydalis Yanhusuo (*Yan Hu Suo*) should be:
    a. Decocted first
    b. Decocted with the other medicinals as usual
    c. Decocted after
    d. Dissolved in the strained decoction
    e. Steeped

    Answer: ___

258. Which of the following medicinals quickens the blood and dispels stasis, disinhibits the gallbladder and recedes or abates jaundice:
    a. Rhizoma Sparganii (*San Leng*)
    b. Tuber Curcumae (*Yu Jin*)
    c. Radix Ligustici Wallichii (*Chuan Xiong*)
    d. Resina Myrrhae (*Mo Yao*)
    e. Resina Olibani (*Ru Xiang*)

    Answer: ___

259. Which of the following medicinals breaks the blood and rectifies the qi, warms the channels and stops pain, especially shoulder and elbow pain due to wind cold damp impediment:
    a. Radix Ligustici Wallichii (*Chuan Xiong*)
    b. Flos Carthami Tinctorii (*Hong Hua*)
    c. Rhizoma Curcumae Longae (*Jiang Huang*)
    d. Rhizoma Sparganii (*San Leng*)
    e. Rhizoma Curcumae Zedoariae (*E Zhu*)

    Answer: ___

260. Which of the following statements is wrong:
    a. Rhizoma Sparganii (*San Leng*) should be decocted first
    b. Feces Trogopterori Seu Pteromi (*Wu Ling Zhi*) should be wrapped during decoction
    c. Gelatinum Corii Asini (*E Jiao*) should be dissolved in the strained decoction
    d. Pyritum (*Zi Ran Tong*) should be ground into fine powder
    e. Tabanus (*Meng Chong*) should be ground into powder

    Answer: ___

261. Which of the following medicinals is best for blood heat painful menstruation or postpartum abdominal pain:
    a. Radix Ligustici Wallichii (*Chuan Xiong*)
    b. Feces Trogopterori Seu Pteromi (*Wu Ling Zhi*)
    c. Radix Salviae Miltiorrhizae (*Dan Shen*)
    d. Rhizoma Curcumae Longae (*Jiang Huang*)
    e. Resina Olibani (*Ru Xiang*)

    Answer: ___

262. Herba Leonuri Heterophylli (*Yi Mu Cao*) is mainly used for:
    a. Blood stasis in gynecology
    b. Blood stasis in internal medicine
    c. Blood stasis in traumatic injury
    d. None of the above
    e. All of the above

    Answer: ___

263. Which of the following medicinals can supplement and move the blood, soothe the sinews and free the flow of the network vessels:
   a. Radix Angelicae Sinensis (*Dang Gui*)
   b. Gelatinum Corii Asini (*E Jiao*)
   c. Caulis Milletiae Seu Spatholobi (*Ji Xue Teng*)
   d. Lignum Sappan (*Su Mu*)
   e. Radix Ligustici Wallichii (*Chuan Xiong*)

   Answer: ___

264. Which of the following medicinals is best for blood stasis abdominal pain and constipation:
   a. Radix Ligustici Wallichii (*Chuan Xiong*)
   b. Tuber Curcumae (*Yu Jin*)
   c. Resina Olibani (*Ru Xiang*)
   d. Flos Carthami Tinctorii (*Hong Hua*)
   e. Semen Pruni Persicae (*Tao Ren*)

   Answer: ___

265. Radix Achyranthis Bidentatae (*Niu Xi*) treats all of the following except:
   a. Painful menstruation, blocked menstruation, and postpartum abdominal pain due to blood stasis
   b. Low back and knee soreness and weakness
   c. Hematuria, dysuria, and painful urination
   d. Hemoptysis, hacking of blood, toothache, and sores in the mouth
   e. Scrofulous lumps and plum pit qi

   Answer: ___

266. Which of the following medicinals quickens the blood, promotes menstruation, promotes lactation, reduces swelling, and discharges pus:
   a. Semen Vaccariae Segetalis (*Wang Bu Liu Xing*)
   b. Radix Echinposis Seu Rhapontici (*Lou Lu*)
   c. Squama Manitis Pentadactylis (*Chuan Shan Jia*)
   d. Radix Platycodi Grandiflori (*Jie Geng*)
   e. Radix Achyranthis Bidentatae (*Niu Xi*)

   Answer: ___

267. Which of the following medicinals A) knits the sinews and bones and B) breaks the blood and dispels stasis:
   a. Radix Dipsaci (*Xu Duan*)
   b. Fructus Psoraleae Corylifoliae (*Bu Gu Zhi*)
   c. Eupolyphaga Seu Opisthoplatia (*Tu Bie Chong*, a.k.a. *Di Bie Chong* & *Zhe Chong*)
   d. Rhizoma Drynariae (*Gu Sui Bu*)
   e. Tabanus (*Meng Chong*)

   Answer: ___

268. Which of the following pairs of medicinals treats agalactia due to blood stasis:
    a. Caulis Akebiae (*Mu Tong*) & Radix Ligustici Wallichii (*Chuan Xiong*)
    b. Radix Ligustici Wallichii (*Chuan Xiong*) & Squama Manitis Pentadactylis (*Chuan Shan Jia*)
    c. Squama Manitis Pentadactylis (*Chuan Shan Jia*) & Semen Vaccariae Segetalis (*Wang Bu Liu Xing*)
    d. Semen Vaccariae Segetalis (*Wang Bu Liu Xing*) & Herba Lycopi Lucidi (*Ze Lan*)
    e. Herba Lycopi Lucidi (*Ze Lan*) & Radix Achyranthis Bidentatae (*Niu Xi*)

    Answer: ___

269. Which of the following medicinals guides the blood to move downward:
    a. Radix Achyranthis Bidentatae (*Niu Xi*)
    b. Flos Carthami Tinctorii (*Hong Hua*)
    c. Radix Salviae Miltiorrhizae (*Dan Shen*)
    d. Radix Ligustici Wallichii (*Chuan Xiong*)
    e. Radix Angelicae Sinensis (*Dang Gui*)

    Answer: ___

270. When used to quicken the blood and stop pain, Feces Trogopterori Seu Pteromi (*Wu Ling Zhi*) is often combined with:
    a. Radix Rubiae Cordifoliae (*Qian Cao Gen*)
    b. Flos Carthami Tinctorii (*Hong Hua*)
    c. Pollen Typhae (*Pu Huang*)
    d. Radix Glycyrrhizae (*Gan Cao*)
    e. Radix Albus Paeoniae Lactiflorae (*Bai Shao*)

    Answer: ___

271. The functions of Tuber Curcumae (*Yu Jin*) are to:
    a. Quicken the blood and rectify the qi, disperse swelling and stop pain
    b. Quicken the blood and rectify the qi, cool the blood and clear heat
    c. Quicken the blood and rectify the qi, dispel wind and stop pain
    d. Quicken the blood and rectify the qi, nourish the blood and quiet the spirit
    e. Quicken the blood and rectify the qi, recede or abate jaundice and quiet the fetus

    Answer: ___

272. The functions of Semen Pruni Persicae (*Tao Ren*) are to:
    a. Move the blood, supplement the blood, and soothe the sinews
    b. Quicken the blood and stop pain, clear heat and eliminate dampness
    c. Quicken the blood and dispel stasis, moisten the intestines and free the flow of the stool
    d. Quicken the blood and stop pain, disperse swelling and disperse stagnation
    e. None of the above

    Answer: ___

Interior-warming Medicinals (*Wen Li Yao*)

273. Interior-warming medicinals do all the following except:
    a. Warm the middle
    b. Fortify the spleen
    c. Scatter cold and stop pain
    d. Invigorate fire to supplement yang
    e. Nourish yin to supplement yang

    Answer: ___

274. Radix Lateralis Praeparatus Aconiti Carmichaeli (*Fu Zi*) invigorates the yang of the:
    a. Heart, liver, and kidneys
    b. Heart, spleen, and kidneys
    c. Spleen, stomach, and kidneys
    d. Spleen, stomach, and bladder
    e. Liver, spleen, and kidneys

    Answer: ___

275. Radix Lateralis Praeparatus Aconiti Carmichaeli (*Fu Zi*) is safer to use when it is boiled for:
    a. A very short time
    b. A long time
    c. Not at all

    Answer: ___

276. When Radix Lateralis Praeparatus Aconiti Carmichaeli (*Fu Zi*) is used to return yang and stem desertion, it is commonly combined with:
    a. Fructus Evodiae Rutecarpae (*Wu Zhu Yu*)
    b. Ramulus Cinnamomi Cassiae (*Gui Zhi*)
    c. Cortex Cinnamomi Cassiae (*Rou Gui*)
    d. uncooked Rhizoma Zingiberis (*Sheng Jiang*)
    e. dry Rhizoma Zingiberis (*Gan Jiang*)

    Answer: ___

277. Radix Lateralis Praeparatus Aconiti Carmichaeli (*Fu Zi*) treats all the following except:
    a. Profuse perspiration due to yang desertion
    b. Aversion to cold and chilled extremities due to yang vacuity
    c. Spontaneous perspiration due to defensive qi vacuity
    d. Cold damp impediment conditions
    e. Dampness and turbidity obstructing the middle burner

    Answer: ___

278. Radix Lateralis Praeparatus Aconiti Carmichaeli (*Fu Zi*) warms _____ yang:
    a. Kidney
    b. Spleen
    c. Heart
    d. whole body's
    e. Lung

    Answer: ___

279. Fructus Foeniculi Vulgaris (*Xiao Hui Xiang*) and Semen Litchi Sinensis (*Li Zhi He*) are often paired to treat:
    a. Damp heat in the lower burner
    b. Damp heat in the liver channel
    c. Cold dampness in the liver channel
    d. Wind cold damp impediment in the lower extremities
    e. Vacuity cold vaginal discharge

    Answer: ___

280. Which of the following medicinals is acrid and hot:
    a. uncooked Rhizoma Zingiberis (*Sheng Jiang*)
    b. Cortex Rhizomatis Zingiberis (*Sheng Jiang Pi*)
    c. dry Rhizoma Zingiberis (*Gan Jiang*)
    d. blast-fried Rhizoma Zingiberis (*Pao Jiang*)
    e. All of the above

    Answer: ___

281. Which of the following medicinals A) warms the middle and returns yang and B) warms the lungs and transforms phlegm:
    a. Radix Lateralis Praeparatus Aconiti Carmichaeli (*Fu Zi*)
    b. Semen Sinapis Albae (*Bai Jie Zi*)
    c. dry Rhizoma Zingiberis (*Gan Jiang*)
    d. Rhizoma Alpiniae Officinari (*Gao Liang Jiang*)
    e. Herba Asari Cum Radice (*Xi Xin*)

    Answer: ___

282. Blast-fried Rhizoma Zingiberis (*Pao Jiang*) is best for:
    a. Warming the middle and scattering cold
    b. Warming the stomach and stopping vomiting
    c. Warming the lungs and transforming phlegm
    d. Warming the channels and stopping bleeding
    e. All of the above

    Answer: ___

283. Dry Rhizoma Zingiberis (*Gan Jiang*) gathers in or enters which "channels":
    a. Spleen & liver
    b. Spleen, stomach, heart & lung
    c. Spleen & stomach
    d. Spleen
    e. Spleen & lung

    Answer: ___

284. Which of the following medicinals is commonly used for cold stagnating in the liver channel qi mounting lower abdominal pain:
    a. Radix Auklandiae Lappae (*Mu Xiang*)
    b. Fructus Evodiae Rutecarpae (*Wu Zhu Yu*)
    c. Fructus Meliae Toosendan (*Chuan Lian Zi*)
    d. dry Rhizoma Zingiberis (*Gan Jiang*)
    e. Rhizoma Corydalis Yanhusuo (*Yan Hu Suo*)

    Answer: ___

285. Cortex Cinnamomi Cassiae (*Rou Gui*)'s functions are to:
    a. Warm the middle, stop pain, and fortify the spleen
    b. Warm the middle, downbear counterflow, and warm the kidneys
    c. Return yang, supplement lifegate fire, scatter cold, and stop pain
    d. Warm the middle, return yang, warm the lungs, and transform phlegm
    e. Supplement lifegate fire, scatter cold, stop pain, and warm the channels and vessels

    Answer: ___

286. Which of the following medicinal is acrid, sweet, and hot and is often used to treat lower burner vacuity cold:
    a. Ramulus Cinnamomi Cassiae (*Gui Zhi*)
    b. Cortex Cinnamomi Cassiae (*Rou Gui*)
    c. Radix Lateralis Praeparatus Aconiti Carmichaeli (*Fu Zi*)
    d. dry Rhizoma Zingiberis (*Gan Jiang*)
    e. Fructus Evodiae Rutecarpae (*Wu Zhu Yu*)

    Answer: ___

287. Herba Asari Cum Radice (*Xi Xin*) treats all of the following except:
    a. Yin vacuity/yang hyperactivity headache
    b. Wind damp impediment conditions
    c. Exterior contraction wind cold headache
    d. Nasal congestion
    e. External contraction wind cold cough with chilly rheum

    Answer: ___

288. Which of the following medicinals A) warms the lungs and transforms cold and B) opens the nasal orifices:
  a. dry Rhizoma Zingiberis (*Gan Jiang*)
  b. Fructus Xanthii Sibirici (*Cang Er Zi*)
  c. Flos Magnoliae Liliflorae (*Xin Yi Hua*)
  d. Herba Asari Cum Radice (*Xi Xin*)
  e. Radix Angelicae Dahuricae (*Bai Zhi*)

  Answer: ___

289. Which of the following medicinals is best for treating a *shao yin* headache:
  a. Radix Et Rhizoma Notopterygii (*Qiang Huo*)
  b. Radix Bupleuri (*Chai Hu*)
  c. Herba Asari Cum Radice (*Xi Xin*)
  d. Radix Angelicae Dahuricae (*Bai Zhi*)
  e. Radix Et Rhizoma Ligustici Chinensis (*Gao Ben*, a.k.a. *Hao Ben*)

  Answer: ___

290. Which of the following medicinals scatters cold and stops pain as well as soothes the liver:
  a. Cortex Cinnamomi Cassiae (*Rou Gui*)
  b. Fructus Evodiae Rutecarpae (*Wu Zhu Yu*)
  c. Fructus Corni Officinalis (*Shan Zhu Yu*)
  d. Fructus Zanthoxyli Bungeani (*Hua Jiao*)
  e. Radix Bupleuri (*Chai Hu*)

  Answer: ___

291. Fructus Evodiae Rutecarpae (*Wu Zhu Yu*) is best for treating which kind of headache:
  a. *Shao yin*
  b. *Jue yin*
  c. *Tai yang*
  d. *Yang ming*
  e. *Shao yang*

  Answer: ___

292. When Fructus Evodiae Rutecarpae (*Wu Zhu Yu*) is used to treat lower abdominal cold stagnating in the liver channel pain, it is usually combined with:
  a. Radix Auklandiae Lappae (*Mu Xiang*) & Rhizoma Cyperi Rotundi (*Xiang Fu*)
  b. Fructus Foeniculi Vulgaris (*Xiao Hui Xiang*) & Radix Linderae Strychnifoliae (*Wu Yao*)
  c. Radix Panacis Ginseng (*Ren Shen*) & uncooked Rhizoma Zingiberis (*Sheng Jiang*)
  d. Semen Myristicae Fragrantis (*Rou Dou Kou*) & Fructus Schisandrae Chinensis (*Wu Wei Zi*)
  e. None of the above

  Answer: ___

293. Which of the following medicinals A) warms the middle and stops pain and B) kills worms:
    a. Fructus Meliae Toosendan (*Chuan Lian Zi*)
    b. Radix Auklandiae Lappae (*Mu Xiang*)
    c. Flos Caryophylli (*Ding Xiang*)
    d. Fructus Cardamomi (*Bai Dou Kou*)
    e. Fructus Zanthoxyli Bungeani (*Hua Jiao*)

    Answer: ___

294. Which of the following medicinals warms the middle, downbears counterflow, and warms kidney yang:
    a. Cortex Magnoliae Officinalis (*Hou Po*)
    b. Pericarpium Citri Reticulatae (*Qing Pi*)
    c. Flos Caryophylli (*Ding Xiang*)
    d. Radix Lateralis Praeparatus Aconiti Carmichaeli (*Fu Zi*)
    e. Fructus Chaenomelis Lagenariae (*Mu Gua*)

    Answer: ___

295. Both dry Rhizoma Zingiberis (*Gan Jiang*) and Rhizoma Alpiniae Officinari (*Gao Liang Jiang*):
    a. Warm the middle and stop pain
    b. Promote sweating and resolve the exterior
    c. Warm the lungs and transform phlegm
    d. Resolve toxins due to fish and shellfish
    e. None of the above

    Answer: ___

296. Which pair of medicinals A) warm the interior and scatter cold and B) course the liver and rectify the qi:
    a. Flos Caryophylli (*Ding Xiang*) & Fructus Evodiae Rutecarpae (*Wu Zhu Yu*)
    b. Fructus Evodiae Rutecarpae (*Wu Zhu Yu*) & Fructus Foeniculi Vulgaris (*Xiao Hui Xiang*)
    c. Fructus Foeniculi Vulgaris (*Xiao Hui Xiang*) & Cortex Cinnamomi Cassiae (*Rou Gui*)
    d. Cortex Cinnamomi Cassiae (*Rou Gui*) & Rhizoma Alpiniae Officinari (*Gao Liang Jiang*)
    e. Rhizoma Alpiniae Officinari (*Gao Liang Jiang*) & Flos Caryophylli (*Ding Xiang*)

    Answer: ___

Qi-supplementing Medicinals (*Bu Qi Yao*)

297. What is the difference in clinical use between red and white Radix Panacis Ginseng (*Ren Shen*):
    a. Red Ginseng invigorates yang, while White Ginseng supplements the qi.
    b. Red Ginseng supplements the qi, while White Ginseng invigorates yang.
    c. Red Ginseng enriches yin, while White Ginseng supplements the qi.
    d. Red Ginseng moves the blood, while White Ginseng nourishes the blood.
    e. Red Ginseng warms the center, while White Ginseng clears heat.

    Answer: ___

298. What is the difference in clinical use between Radix Panacis Quinquefolii (*Xi Yang Shen*) and Radix Panacis Ginseng (*Ren Shen*):
    a. Radix Panacis Quinquefolii invigorates yang, while Radix Panacis Ginseng supplements the qi.
    b. Radix Panacis Quinquefolii supplements the qi, while Radix Panacis Ginseng nourishes the blood.
    c. Radix Panacis Quinquefolii nourishes yin, while Radix Panacis Ginseng supplements the qi.
    d. Radix Panacis Quinquefolii dries dampness, while Radix Panacis Ginseng quickens the blood.
    e. Radix Panacis Quinquefolii moves the qi, while Radix Panacis Ginseng moves the blood.

    Answer: ___

299. Radix Panacis Ginseng (*Ren Shen*) is contraindicated in cases of:
    a. Severe spleen qi vacuity
    b. Severe kidney yang vacuity
    c. Severe blood vacuity
    d. Ascendant liver yang hyperactivity
    e. Women

    Answer: ___

300. Radix Panacis Ginseng (*Ren Shen*) supplements all five viscera, while Radix Codonopsitis Pilosulae (*Dang Shen*) only supplements:
    a. Liver & kidneys
    b. Heart & kidneys
    c. Kidneys & spleen
    d. Spleen & liver
    e. Lungs & spleen

    Answer: ___

301. Which of the following medicinals can be used in severe qi desertion with a faint (*wei*) or weak (*rou*) pulse:
    a. Radix Lateralis Praeparatus Aconiti Carmichaeli (*Fu Zi*)
    b. Radix Codonopsitis Pilosulae (*Dang Shen*)
    c. dry Rhizoma Zingiberis (*Gan Jiang*)
    d. Radix Panacis Ginseng (*Ren Shen*)
    e. Radix Astragali Membranacei (*Huang Qi*)

    Answer: ___

302. Which of the following medicinals is often cooked separately in a double boiler for a long period of time:
    a. Fructus Amomi (*Sha Ren*)
    b. Herba Menthae Haplocalycis (*Bo He*)
    c. Radix Panacis Ginseng (*Ren Shen*)
    d. Concha Ostreae (*Mu Li*)
    e. Styrax Liquidus (*Su He Xiang*)

    Answer: ___

303. When Radix Panacis Ginseng (*Ren Shen*) is used to stem desertion, its dosage in decoction should be:
    a. 0.5-1g
    b. 1-3g
    c. 3-6g
    d. 6-9g
    e. 15-30g

    Answer: ___

304. Which medicinal supplements the chest qi more quickly:
    a. Radix Panacis Ginseng (*Ren Shen*)
    b. Radix Astragali Membranacei (*Huang Qi*)

    Answer: ___

305. Which one of these medicinals does not quiet the fetus:
    a. Radix Scutellariae Baicalensis (*Huang Qin*)
    b. Rhizoma Atractylodis Macrocephalae (*Bai Zhu*)
    c. Fructus Amomi (*Sha Ren*)
    d. Radix Codonopsitis Pilosulae (*Dang Shen*)
    e. Cortex Eucommiae Ulmoidis (*Du Zhong*)

    Answer: ___

306. Which is not one of the functions of Radix Glycyrrhizae (*Gan Cao*):
    a. Quickens the blood and transforms stasis
    b. Relaxes tension (spasms or cramps) and stops pain
    c. Clears heat and resolves toxins
    d. Moistens the lungs and stops cough
    e. Supplements the spleen and boosts the qi

    Answer: ___

307. Which of the following medicinals is best for treating qi and fluid vacuity with poor appetite and dry mouth:
    a. Radix Astragali Membranacei (*Huang Qi*)
    b. Rhizoma Atractylodis Macrocephalae (*Bai Zhu*)
    c. Radix Pseudostellariae (*Tai Zi Shen*)
    d. Semen Dolichoris Lablab (*Bai Bian Dou*)
    e. Semen Nelumbinis Nuciferae (*Lian Zi*)

    Answer: ___

308. Which of the following medicinals supplements the qi and upbears yang, secures the exterior and discharges pus:
    a. Rhizoma Cimicifugae (*Sheng Ma*)
    b. Radix Bupleuri (*Chai Hu*)
    c. Radix Astragali Membranacei (*Huang Qi*)
    d. Radix Puerariae (*Ge Gen*)
    e. Radix Codonopsitis Pilosulae (*Dang Shen*)

    Answer: ___

309. Radix Astragali Membranacei (*Huang Qi*) gathers in or enters which "channels":
    a. Spleen & lung
    b. Lung & kidney
    c. Liver & gallbladder
    d. Heart & kidney
    e. All of the above

    Answer: ___

310. Which of the following medicinals fortifies the spleen and supplements the qi, dries dampness, stops sweating, and quiets the fetus:
    a. Radix Dioscoreae Oppositae (*Shan Yao*)
    b. Radix Astragali Membranacei (*Huang Qi*)
    c. Radix Ephedrae (*Ma Huang Gen*)
    d. Sclerotium Poriae Cocos (*Fu Ling*)
    e. Rhizoma Atractylodis Macrocephalae (*Bai Zhu*)

    Answer: ___

311. Which of the following medicinals supplements the spleen and kidneys and treats seminal emission and abnormal vaginal discharge:
    a. Radix Panacis Ginseng (*Ren Shen*)
    b. Radix Codonopsitis Pilosulae (*Dang Shen*)
    c. Radix Astragali Membranacei (*Huang Qi*)
    d. Radix Dioscoreae Oppositae (*Shan Yao*)
    e. Semen Astragali Complanati (*Sha Yuan Zi*)

    Answer: ___

312. Radix Dioscoreae Oppositae (*Shan Yao*)'s functions are to:
    a. Fortify the spleen and supplement the qi, supplement the lungs and stop cough
    b. Supplement the lungs and kidneys, supplement the qi and enrich yin
    c. Supplement the qi and enrich yin, fortify the spleen and supplement the lungs and kidneys
    d. Supplement the kidneys and enrich yin, fortify the spleen and boost the stomach
    e. Cool the blood and nourish yin, supplement the lungs, spleen, and kidneys

    Answer: ___

313. Which of the following medicinals can supplement the middle and relax tension (cramps or spasms), moisten the lungs and stop cough, moisten the intestines and free the flow of the stools:
    a. Semen Cannabis Sativae (*Huo Ma Ren*)
    b. Semen Pruni (*Yu Li Ren*)
    c. Mel (*Feng Mi, i.e.*, honey)
    d. Herba Cistanchis Deserticolae (*Rou Cong Rong*)
    e. Radix Angelicae Sinensis (*Dang Gui*)

    Answer: ___

314. Both Radix Dioscoreae Oppositae (*Shan Yao*) and Semen Dolichoris Lablab (*Bai Bian Dou*):
    a. Harmonize the middle and dry dampness
    b. Fortify the spleen and stop diarrhea
    c. Supplement the kidneys and secure and astringe
    d. Supplement the qi and enrich yin
    e. Engender fluids and stop thirst

    Answer: ___

Blood-supplementing Medicinals (*Bu Xue Yao*)

315. The standard modern dose of cooked Radix Rehmanniae (*Shu Di*) is:
    a. 4.5-12g
    b. 6-15g
    c. 9-30g
    d. 1.5-4.5g

    Answer: ___

316. Which form of Rehmannia (*Di Huang*) is more glossy and enriching and, therefore, more likely to cause diarrhea:
    a. uncooked Radix Rehmanniae (*Sheng Di*)
    b. cooked Radix Rehmanniae (*Shu Di*)

    Answer: ___

317. To supplement the blood, combine cooked Radix Rehmanniae (*Shu Di*) with:
    a. Radix Bupleuri (*Chai Hu*)
    b. Radix Auklandiae Lappae (*Mu Xiang*)
    c. Pericarpium Citri Reticulatae (*Chen Pi*)
    d. Radix Angelicae Sinensis (*Dang Gui*)
    e. Folium Perillae Frutescentis (*Zi Su Ye*)

    Answer: ___

318. Which blood supplement also secures the essence and stops leakage:
    a. Radix Angelicae Sinensis (*Dang Gui*)
    b. Radix Polygoni Multiflori (*He Shou Wu*)
    c. Caulis Milletiae Seu Spatholobi (*Ji Xue Teng*)
    d. Gelatinum Corii Asini (*E Jiao*)
    e. Fructus Lycii Chinensis (*Gou Qi Zi*)

    Answer: ___

319. Radix Albus Paeoniae Lactiflorae (*Bai Shao*) gathers in or enters which "channels":
    a. Liver & heart
    b. Liver & large intestines
    c. Liver & spleen
    d. Liver & kidneys
    e. Kidneys & heart

    Answer: ___

320. In order to relax tension, spasms, or cramps, Radix Albus Paeoniae Lactiflorae (*Bai Shao*) is usually combined with:
    a. Fructus Zizyphi Jujubae (*Da Zao*)
    b. Radix Codonopsitis Pilosulae (*Dang Shen*)
    c. Radix Angelicae Sinensis (*Dang Gui*)
    d. Caulis Milletiae Seu Spatholobi (*Ji Xue Teng*)
    e. Radix Glycyrrhizae (*Gan Cao*)

    Answer: ___

321. Which is the best blood supplement for boosting the essence and brightening the eyes:
    a. Fructus Lycii Chinensis (*Gou Qi Zi*)
    b. Radix Angelicae Sinensis (*Dang Gui*)
    c. Radix Albus Paeoniae Lactiflorae (*Bai Shao*)
    d. cooked Radix Rehmanniae (*Shu Di*)
    e. Gelatinum Corii Asini (*E Jiao*)

    Answer: ___

322. Which of the following medicinals can be used for blood vacuity, blood cold, and blood stasis:
    a. cooked Radix Rehmanniae (*Shu Di*)
    b. Radix Polygoni Multiflori (*He Shou Wu*)
    c. Gelatinum Corii Asini (*E Jiao*)
    d. Radix Albus Paeoniae Lactiflorae (*Bai Shao*)
    e. Radix Angelicae Sinensis (*Dang Gui*)

    Answer: ___

323. Which of the following medicinals supplement the blood and regulates menstruation, moistens the intestines and frees the flow of the stools:
    a. Radix Polygoni Multiflori (*He Shou Wu*)
    b. Radix Angelicae Sinensis (*Dang Gui*)
    c. Arillus Euphoriae Longanae (*Long Yan Rou*)
    d. Gelatinum Corii Asini (*E Jiao*)
    e. cooked Radix Rehmanniae (*Shu Di*)

    Answer: ___

324. Stir-frying Radix Angelicae Sinensis (*Dang Gui*) increases its ability to:
    a. Supplement the blood
    b. Moisten the intestines
    c. Quicken the blood
    d. All of the above
    e. None of the above

    Answer: ___

325. Cooked Radix Rehmanniae (*Shu Di*)'s functions are to:
 a. Supplement the qi and nourish the blood
 b. Nourish the blood and enrich yin
 c. Nourish yin and cool the blood
 d. Cool and quicken the blood
 e. Nourish and break the blood

Answer: ___

326. Which of the following medicinals can be used to treat A) a sallow yellow facial complexion, heart palpitations, and insomnia due to blood vacuity and B) tidal emission of heat, night sweats, dizziness, and tinnitus due to kidney yin vacuity:
 a. Fructus Corni Officinalis (*Shan Zhu Yu*)
 b. Rhizoma Anemarrhenae Aspheloidis (*Zhi Mu*)
 c. Radix Angelicae Sinensis (*Dang Gui*)
 d. cooked Radix Rehmanniae (*Shu Di*)
 e. Semen Zizyphi Spinosae (*Suan Zao Ren*)

Answer: ___

327. Which of the following medicinals A) resolves toxins and moistens the intestines when used uncooked and B) supplements the blood and boosts the essence when used processed:
 a. Herba Cistanchis Deserticolae (*Rou Cong Rong*)
 b. Radix Lithospermi Seu Arnebiae (*Zi Cao*)
 c. Radix Polygoni Multiflori (*He Shou Wu*)
 d. Radix Achyranthis Bidentatae (*Niu Xi*)
 e. Radix Astragali Membranacei (*Huang Qi*)

Answer: ___

328. Which of the following medicinals A) nourishes the blood and astringes yin and B) subdues liver yang:
 a. Radix Albus Paeoniae Lactiflorae (*Bai Shao*)
 b. Flos Chrysanthemi Morifolii (*Ju Hua*)
 c. Concha Haliotidis (*Shi Jue Ming*)
 d. Semen Cassiae Torae (*Jue Ming Zi*)
 e. cooked Radix Rehmanniae (*Shu Di*)

Answer: ___

329. Which of the following medicinals astringe yin, harmonize the constructive, and stop sweating:
 a. Concha Ostreae (*Mu Li*)
 b. Radix Ephedrae (*Ma Huang Gen*)
 c. Radix Astragali Membranacei (*Huang Qi*)
 d. Radix Albus Paeoniae Lactiflorae (*Bai Shao*)
 e. Rhizoma Atractylodis Macrocephalae (*Bai Zhu*)

Answer: ___

330. Which of the following medicinals A) supplements the blood and stops bleeding and B) enriches yin and moistens the lungs:
    a. Rhizoma Polygonati Odorati (*Yu Zhu*)
    b. Tuber Asparagi Cochinensis (*Tian Men Dong*)
    c. Rhizoma Polygonati (*Huang Jing*)
    d. Gelatinum Corii Asini (*E Jiao*)
    e. Radix Angelicae Sinensis (*Dang Gui*)

    Answer: ___

331. Arillus Euphoriae Longanae (*Long Yan Rou*)'s functions are to:
    a. Supplement the heat and spleen, boost the qi and nourish the blood
    b. Supplement the lungs and spleen, quiet the spirit
    c. Supplement the lungs and kidneys, level panting
    d. Supplement the spleen and kidneys, stop diarrhea
    e. Supplement the liver and kidneys, brighten the eyes

    Answer: ___

Yang-supplementing Medicinals (*Bu Yang Yao*)

332. Most yang supplements also:
    a. Nourish liver blood
    b. Supplement heart qi
    c. Supplement spleen qi
    d. Engender fluids
    e. Rectify the qi

    Answer: ___

333. Which of the following medicinals A) supplements the kidneys and invigorates yang and B) moistens the intestines and frees the flow of the stools:
    a. Fructus Psoraleae Corylifoliae (*Bu Gu Zhi*)
    b. Semen Trigonellae Foeni-graeci (*Hu Lu Ba*)
    c. Herba Cistanchis Deserticolae (*Rou Cong Rong*)
    d. Cornu Degelatinum Cervi (*Lu Jiao Shuang*)
    e. Radix Morindae Officinalis (*Ba Ji Tian*)

    Answer: ___

334. Cortex Eucommiae Ulmoidis (*Du Zhong*)'s flavor and nature (*i.e.*, temperature) are:
    a. Acrid & warm
    b. Bitter & warm
    c. Sweet & warm
    d. Salty & warm
    e. Sour & warm

    Answer: ___

335. Cortex Eucommiae Ulmoidis (*Du Zhong*)'s functions are to:
    a. Supplement the liver and kidneys, secure the essence and brighten the eyes
    b. Supplement the liver and kidneys, strengthen the sinews and bones, quiet the fetus
    c. Supplement the liver and kidneys, nourish the blood and fill the essence
    d. Supplement the liver and kidneys, guide the blood to move downward
    e. Supplement the liver and kidneys, warm the uterus and stop bleeding

    Answer: ___

336. Which of the following medicinals A) supplements the liver and kidneys and B) quickens the blood and strengthens the sinews and bones:
    a. Ramulus Loranthi Seu Visci (*Sang Ji Sheng*)
    b. Radix Achyranthis Bidentatae (*Niu Xi*)
    c. Radix Dipsaci (*Xu Duan*)
    d. Radix Morindae Officinalis (*Ba Ji Tian*)
    e. Semen Trigonellae Foeni-graeci (*Hu Lu Ba*)

    Answer: ___

337. Which of the following medicinals treats enduring diarrhea due to spleen-kidney dual vacuity:
    a. Radix Puerariae (*Ge Gen*)
    b. Fructus Psoraleae Corylifoliae (*Bu Gu Zhi*)
    c. Semen Myristicae Fragrantis (*Rou Dou Kou*)
    d. Semen Nelumbinis Nuciferae (*Lian Zi*)
    e. Fructus Schisandrae Chinensis (*Wu Wei Zi*)

    Answer: ___

338. Which of the following medicinals supplements the kidneys, secures the essence, warms the spleen, and treats excessively profuse saliva:
    a. Fructus Alpiniae Oxyphyllae (*Yi Zhi Ren*)
    b. Fructus Rubi Chingii (*Fu Pen Zi*)
    c. Semen Astragali Complanati (*Sha Yuan Zi*)
    d. Fructus Schisandrae Chinensis (*Wu Wei Zi*)
    e. Fructus Psoraleae Corylifoliae (*Bu Gu Zhi*)

    Answer: ___

339. Cordyceps (*Dong Chong Xia Cao*)'s functions are to:
    a. Supplement the liver and kidneys
    b. Supplement the spleen and kidneys
    c. Supplement the lungs and kidneys
    d. Supplement the heart and liver
    e. Supplement the heart and spleen

    Answer: ___

340. Which of the following medicinals supplements yang and nourishes yin, secures the essence and astringes urination, brightens the eyes and stops diarrhea:
    a. Placenta Hominis (*Zi He Che*)
    b. Radix Morindae Officinalis (*Ba Ji Tian*)
    c. Semen Astragali Complanati (*Sha Yuan Zi*)
    d. Semen Cuscutae Chinensis (*Tu Si Zi*)
    e. Semen Trigonellae Foeni-graeci (*Hu Lu Ba*)

    Answer: ___

341. Which pair of yang-supplementing medicinals is best to treat yang vacuity premature ovarian decline and lack of or decreased libido:
    a. Radix Dipsaci (*Xu Duan*) & Cortex Eucommiae Ulmoidis (*Du Zhong*)
    b. Herba Epimedii (*Xian Ling Pi*) & Rhizoma Curculiginis Orchioidis (*Xian Mao*)
    c. Herba Cistanchis Deserticolae (*Rou Cong Rong*) & Radix Angelicae Sinensis (*Dang Gui*)
    d. Fructus Psoraleae Corylifoliae (*Bu Gu Zhi*) & Semen Cuscutae Chinensis (*Tu Si Zi*)
    e. Semen Alpiniae Oxyphyllae (*Yi Zhi Ren*) & Rhizoma Acori Graminei (*Shi Chang Pu*)

    Answer: ___

342. Which pair of yang-supplementing medicinals is best to treat kidney yang vacuity low back and knee soreness and weakness:
    a. Radix Dipsaci (*Xu Duan*) & Cortex Eucommiae Ulmoidis (*Du Zhong*)
    b. Herba Epimedii (*Xian Ling Pi*) & Rhizoma Curculiginis Orchioidis (*Xian Mao*)
    c. Herba Cistanchis Deserticolae (*Rou Cong Rong*) & Radix Angelicae Sinensis (*Dang Gui*)
    d. Fructus Psoraleae Corylifoliae (*Bu Gu Zhi*) & Semen Cuscutae Chinensis (*Tu Si Zi*)
    e. Semen Alpiniae Oxyphyllae (*Yi Zhi Ren*) & Rhizoma Acori Graminei (*Shi Chang Pu*)

    Answer: ___

Yin-supplementing Medicinals (*Bu Yin Yao*)

343. Bulbus Lilii (*Bai He*) gathers in or enters which "channels":
    a. Heart & kidneys
    b. Heart & spleen
    c. Heart & lungs
    d. Heart & small intestines
    e. Heart & liver

    Answer: ___

344. Which yin supplement also quickens the blood:
    a. Fructus Ligustri Lucidi (*Nu Zhen Zi*)
    b. Carapax Amydae Sinensis (*Bei Jia*)
    c. Herba Ecliptae Prostratae (*Han Lian Cao*)
    d. Ramulus Loranthi Seu Visci (*Sang Ji Sheng*)
    e. Bulbus Lilii (*Bai He*)

    Answer: ___

345. Which of the following medicinals not only nourishes lung and stomach yin but also clears lung and stomach heat:
    a. Gypsum Fibrosum (*Shi Gao*)
    b. Folium Lophatheri Gracilis (*Dan Zhu Ye*)
    c. Fructus Lycii Chinensis (*Gou Qi Zi*)
    d. Radix Scutellariae Baicalensis (*Huang Qin*)
    e. Radix Glehniae Littoralis (*Sha Shen*)

    Answer: ___

346. Which of the following medicinals should be used to treat vexation, insomnia, and heart palpitations due to heart yin vacuity:
    a. Folium Lophatheri Gracilis (*Dan Zhu Ye*)
    b. Tuber Ophiopogonis Japonici (*Mai Men Dong*)
    c. Rhizoma Coptidis Chinensis (*Huang Lian*)
    d. Plumula Nelumbinis Nuciferae (*Lian Zi Xin*)
    e. Fructus Gardeniae Jasminoidis (*Shan Zhi Zi*)

    Answer: ___

347. Which of the following medicinals is best for stomach yin vacuity:
    a. Radix Glehniae Littoralis (*Sha Shen*)
    b. Rhizoma Polygonati (*Huang Jing*)
    c. Herba Dendrobii (*Shi Hu*)
    d. Tuber Ophiopogonis Japonici (*Mai Men Dong*)
    e. Bulbus Lilii (*Bai He*)

    Answer: ___

348. Which of the following medicinals not only nourishes stomach yin and engenders fluids but also enriches kidney yin and clears vacuity heat:
    a. Tuber Asparagi Cochinensis (*Tian Men Dong*)
    b. Tuber Ophiopogonis Japonici (*Mai Men Dong*)
    c. Radix Glehniae Littoralis (*Sha Shen*)
    d. Herba Dendrobii (*Shi Hu*)
    e. Rhizoma Polygonati Odorati (*Yu Zhu*)

    Answer: ___

349. Which of the following medicinals A) supplements the spleen and boosts the qi and B) moistens the lungs and nourishes yin:
    a. Radix Glycyrrhizae (*Gan Cao*)
    b. Rhizoma Polygonati (*Huang Jing*)
    c. Rhizoma Polygonati Odorati (*Yu Zhu*)
    d. Radix Astragali Membranacei (*Huang Qi*)
    e. Herba Dendrobii (*Shi Hu*)

    Answer: ___

350. Which of the following medicinals A) clears the heart and quiets the spirit and B) moistens the lungs and stops cough:
    a. Bulbus Lilii (*Bai He*)
    b. Radix Salviae Miltiorrhizae (*Dan Shen*)
    c. Bulbus Fritillariae Cirrhosae (*Chuan Bei Mu*)
    d. Radix Glehniae Littoralis (*Sha Shen*)
    e. Rhizoma Coptidis Chinensis (*Huang Lian*)

    Answer: ___

351. Which of the following medicinals is best to treat decrease in visual acuity due to liver-kidney vacuity:
    a. Concha Haliotidis (*Shi Jue Ming*)
    b. Semen Cassiae Torae (*Jue Ming Zi*)
    c. Fructus Lycii Chinensis (*Gou Qi Zi*)
    d. Ramulus Loranthi Seu Visci (*Sang Ji Sheng*)
    e. Fructus Viticis (*Man Jing Zi*)

    Answer: ___

352. All of the following medicinals clear the lungs and engender fluids. Which one also supplements the kidneys and enriches yin:
    a. Radix Glehniae Littoralis (*Sha Shen*)
    b. Tuber Ophiopogonis Japonici (*Mai Men Dong*)
    c. Rhizoma Phragmitis Communis (*Lu Gen*)
    d. Radix Trichosanthis Kirlowii (*Tian Hua Fen*)
    e. Tuber Asparagi Cochinensis (*Tian Men Dong*)

    Answer: ___

353. Both Rhizoma Polygonati Odorati (*Yu Zhu*) and Radix Glehniae Littoralis (*Sha Shen*):
  a. Supplement liver and kidney yin
  b. Clear heart and lung heat
  c. Nourish lung and stomach yin
  d. Drain liver and gallbladder fire
  e. None of the above

  Answer: ___

354. Which pair of medicinals nourishes the blood and enriches yin without being slimy and stagnating:
  a. cooked Radix Rehmanniae (*Shu Di*) & uncooked Radix Rehmanniae (*Sheng Di*)
  b. Radix Polygoni Multiflori (*He Shou Wu*) & Radix Angelicae Sinensis (*Dang Gui*)
  c. Fructus Ligustri Lucidi (*Nu Zhen Zi*) & Herba Ecliptae Prostratae (*Han Lian Cao*)
  d. Gelatinum Corii Asini (*E Jiao*) & Gelatinum Plastri Testudinis (*Gui Ban Jiao*)
  e. Gelatinum Plastri Testudinis (*Gui Ban Jiao*) & Gelatinum Cornu Cervi (*Lu Jiao Jiao*)

  Answer: ___

Astringing & Securing Medicinals (*Se Gu Yao*)

355. Which astringent medicinal A) secures and astringes the intestines, B) warms the middle, and C) moves the qi:
    a. Pericarpium Punicae Granati (*Shi Liu Pi*)
    b. Fructus Pruni Mume (*Wu Mei*)
    c. Semen Myristicae Fragrantis (*Rou Dou Kou*)
    d. Fructus Terminaliae Chebulae (*He Zi*)
    e. Semen Euryalis Ferocis (*Qian Shi*)

    Answer: ___

356. Which astringent medicinal supplements the spleen, kidneys, and heart:
    a. Semen Euryalis Ferocis (*Qian Shi*)
    b. Fructus Pruni Mume (*Wu Mei*)
    c. Cortex Ailanthi Altissimi (*Chun Gen Pi*)
    d. Semen Nelumbinis Nuciferae (*Lian Zi*)
    e. Pericarpium Papaveris Somniferi (*Ying Su Ke*)

    Answer: ___

357. Which astringent medicinal supplements the spleen, secures the kidneys, and dispels dampness:
    a. Semen Euryalis Ferocis (*Qian Shi*)
    b. Fructus Schisandrae Chinensis (*Wu Wei Zi*)
    c. Fructus Rosae Laevigatae (*Jin Ying Zi*)
    d. Pericarpium Puinicae Granati (*Shi Liu Pi*)
    e. Cortex Ailanthi Altissimi (*Chun Gen Pi*)

    Answer: ___

358. Which of the following medicinals A) supplements the spleen and stops diarrhea and B) supplements the kidneys and secures the essence:
    a. Fructus Rosae Laevigatae (*Jin Ying Zi*)
    b. Fructus Terminaliae Chebulae (*He Zi*)
    c. Semen Nelumbinis Nuciferae (*Lian Zi*)
    d. Fructus Pruni Mume (*Wu Mei*)
    e. Cortex Ailanthi Altissimi (*Chun Gen Pi*)

    Answer: ___

359. Which of the following medicinals supplements the liver and kidneys and secures and astringes:
    a. Fructus Corni Officinalis (*Shan Zhu Yu*)
    b. Herba Ecliptae Prostratae (*Han Lian Cao*)
    c. Semen Astragali Complanati (*Sha Yuan Zi*)
    d. Fructus Ligustri Lucidi (*Nu Zhen Zi*)
    e. Fructus Mori Albi (*Sang Shen*)

    Answer: ___

360. Which set of medicinals secures the intestines and stops diarrhea:
   a. Fructus Terminaliae Chebulae (*He Zi*), Fructus Schisandrae Chinensis (*Wu Wei Zi*) & Fructus Rubi Chingii (*Fu Pen Zi*)
   b. Hallyositum Rubrum (*Chi Shi Zhi*), Fructus Pruni Mume (*Wu Mei*) & Ootheca Mantidis (*Sang Piao Xiao*)
   c. Galla Rhois (*Wu Bei Zi*) & Fructus Corni Officinalis (*Shan Zhu Yu*)
   d. Semen Myristicae Fragrantis (*Rou Dou Kou*), Pericarpium Papaveris Somniferi (*Ying Su Ke*) & Os Sepiae Seu Sepiellae (*Wu Zei Gu*)
   e. Fructus Terminaliae Chebulae (*He Zi*), Hallyositum Rubrum (*Chi Shi Zhi*) & Semen Myristicae Fragrantis (*Rou Dou Kou*)

   Answer: ___

361. Which pair of medicinals secures the exterior and stops sweating:
   a. Fructus Levis Tritici Aestivi (*Fu Xiao Mai*) & Fructus Rosae Laevigatae (*Jin Ying Zi*)
   b. Radix Ephedrae (*Ma Huang Gen*) & Fructus Pruni Mume (*Wu Mei*)
   c. Fructus Schisandrae Chinensis (*Wu Wei Zi*) & Galla Rhois (*Wu Bei Zi*)
   d. Fructus Levis Tritici Aestivi (*Fu Xiao Mai*) & Pericarpium Punicae Granati *(Shi Liu Pi)*
   e. Fructus Rosae Laevigatae (*Jin Ying Zi*) & Galla Rhois (*Wu Bei Zi*)

   Answer: ___

362. Which pair of medicinals engenders fluids and stops thirst:
   a. Fructus Schisandrae Chinensis (*Wu Wei Zi*) & Fructus Pruni Mume (*Wu Mei*)
   b. Fructus Pruni Mume (*Wu Mei*) & Galla Rhois (*Wu Bei Zi*)
   c. Galla Rhois (*Wu Bei Zi*) & Semen Nelumbinis Nuciferae (*Lian Zi*)
   d. Semen Nelumbinis Nuciferae (*Lian Zi*) & Fructus Corni Officinalis (*Shan Zhu Yu*)
   e. Fructus Corni Officinalis (*Shan Zhu Yu*) & Fructus Schisandrae Chinensis (*Wu Wei Zi*)

   Answer: ___

363. Fructus Schisandrae Chinensis (*Wu Wei Zi*) and Galla Rhois (*Wu Bei Zi*) both:
   a. Supplement the qi and engender fluids
   b. Clear the lungs and drain fire
   c. Secure the lungs and stop sweating
   d. Quiet the spirit
   e. Course the liver and rectify the qi

   Answer: ___

Spirit-quieting Medicinals (*An Shen Yao*)

364. Which heavy spirit-quieting medicinal also softens the hard and scatters nodulations:
    a. Os Draconis (*Long Gu*)
    b. Magnetitum (*Ci Shi*)
    c. Succinum (*Hu Po*)
    d. Concha Ostreae (*Mu Li*)
    e. Margarita (*Zhen Zhu*)

    Answer: ___

365. Os Draconis (*Long Gu*) and Concha Ostreae (*Mu Li*) are usually:
    a. Decocted first
    b. Decocted after
    c. Decocted with the other medicinals
    d. Dissolved in the strained decoction

    Answer: ___

366. Os Draconis (*Long Gu*) and Concha Ostreae (*Mu Li*) are usually used in doses:
    a. Less than 9g
    b. Of 9g
    c. More than 9g
    d. Dose does not matter

    Answer: ___

367. Succinum (*Hu Po*) is usually:
    a. Decocted first
    b. Decocted after
    c. Decocted with the other medicinals
    d. Dissolved in the strained decoction
    e. Chased by the strained decoction

    Answer: ___

368. Succinum (*Hu Po*):
    a. Calms the spirit and stops tetany
    b. Quickens the blood and dispels stasis
    c. Disinhibits urination and frees the flow of strangury
    d. Disperses swelling and heals sores
    e. All of the above

    Answer: ___

369. Haemititum (*Dai Zhe Shi*) levels the liver and subdues yang and:
    a. Cools the blood and stops bleeding
    b. Strongly downbears counterflow
    c. Courses the liver and resolves depression
    d. A & B
    e. B & C

    Answer: ___

370. Which of the following medicinals treats disquietude of the spirit with vexatious heat in the chest, heart palpitations, and insomnia due to heart fire hyperactivity:
    a. Cinnabar (*Zhu Sha*)
    b. Magnetitum (*Ci Shi*)
    c. Sclerotium Pararadicis Poriae Cocos (*Fu Shen*)
    d. Caulis Polygoni Multiflori (*Ye Jiao Teng*)
    e. Folium Lophatheri Gracilis (*Dan Zhu Ye*)

    Answer: ___

371. Magnetitum (*Ci Shi*) treats:
    a. Panting and wheezing due to non-diffusion of lung qi
    b. Panting and wheezing due to lung qi vacuity
    c. Panting and wheezing due to phlegm obstruction
    d. Panting and wheezing due to kidneys not grasping or absorbing
    e. None of the above

    Answer: ___

372. Besides nourishing the heart and quieting the spirit, Semen Zizyphi Spinosae (*Suan Zao Ren*) also:
    a. Courses the liver
    b. Secures the essence
    c. Disinhibits urination
    d. Stops sweating
    e. Quickens the blood

    Answer: ___

373. Which medicinal is best for heart palpitations, insomnia, impaired memory, profuse dreams, and night sweats:
    a. Cinnabar (*Zhu Sha*)
    b. Semen Zizyphi Spinosae (*Suan Zao Ren*)
    c. Semen Biotae Orientalis (*Bai Zi Ren*)
    d. Radix Polygalae Tenuifoliae (*Yuan Zhi*)
    e. Concha Ostreae (*Mu Li*)

    Answer: ___

374. Besides nourishing the heart and quieting the spirit, Semen Biotae Orientalis (*Bai Zi Ren*) also:
    a. Courses the liver
    b. Disinhibits urination
    c. Quickens the blood
    d. Moistens the intestines
    e. Secures the essence

    Answer: ___

375. Which spirit-quieting medicinal also quickens the blood and stops pain:
    a. Cortex Albizziae Julibrissin (*He Huan Pi*)
    b. Caulis Polygoni Multiflori (*Ye Jiao Teng*)
    c. Radix Polygalae Tenuifoliae (*Yuan Zhi*)
    d. Semen Zizyphi Spinosae (*Suan Zao Ren*)
    e. Semen Biotae Orientalis (*Bai Zi Ren*)

    Answer: ___

376. Which of the following medicinals calms the heart and quiets the spirit, transforms phlegm and opens the orifices, disperses swelling and treats welling abscesses:
    a. Calculus Bovis (*Niu Huang*)
    b. Rhizoma Acori Graminei (*Shi Chang Pu*)
    c. Cortex Albizziae Julibrissinis (*He Huan Pi*)
    d. Radix Polygalae Tenuifoliae (*Yuan Zhi*)
    e. Tuber Curcumae (*Yu Jin*)

    Answer: ___

377. Which of the following medicinals is best for profuse dreaming due to heart-liver blood vacuity:
    a. Radix Angelicae Sinensis (*Dang Gui*)
    b. Radix Polygoni Multiflori (*He Shou Wu*)
    c. Caulis Polygoni Multiflori (*Ye Jiao Teng*)
    d. Succinum (*Hu Po*)
    e. Os Draconis (*Long Gu*)

    Answer: ___

378. Which of the following medicinals is best for irritability, emotional depression, insomnia, and impaired memory due to liver depression qi stagnation:
    a. Cortex Albizziae Julibrissinis (*He Huan Pi*)
    b. Caulis Polygoni Multiflori (*Ye Jiao Teng*)
    c. Radix Bupleuri (*Chai Hu*)
    d. Tuber Curcumae (*Yu Jin*)
    e. Fructus Zizyphi Jujubae (*Da Zao*)

    Answer: ___

Wind-extinguishing, Liver-leveling Medicinals (*Xi Feng Ping Gan Yao*)

379. Cornu ___ can be substituted for Cornu Antelopis Saiga-tatarici (*Ling Yang Jiao*):
    a. Cervi (*Lu Jiao*)
    b. Caprae (*Yang Jiao*)
    c. Rhinocerotis (*Xi Jiao*)
    d. Canis (*Kou Jiao*)
    e. Felis (*Miao Jiao*)

    Answer: ___

380. Ramulus Uncariae Cum Uncis (*Gou Teng*) should be:
    a. Decocted first
    b. Decocted after
    c. Decocted with the other medicinals as usual
    d. Dissolved in the strained decoction
    e. Stirred, not shaken

    Answer: ___

381. Rhizoma Gastrodiae Elatae (*Tian Ma*) gathers in or enters which "channel":
    a. Heart
    b. Spleen
    c. Liver
    d. Kidney
    e. Lung

    Answer: ___

382. Which of the following medicinals treats external wind as well as extinguishes liver wind:
    a. Cornu Antelopis Saiga-tatarici (*Ling Yang Jiao*)
    b. Rhizoma Gastrodiae Elatae (*Tian Ma*)
    c. Ramulus Uncariae Cum Uncis (*Gou Teng*)
    d. Lumbricus (*Di Long*)
    e. Radix Bupleuri (*Chai Hu*)

    Answer: ___

383. Which of the following medicinals can be used to stop tetany no matter whether a cold or heat pattern:
    a. Rhizoma Arisaematis (*Tian Nan Xing*)
    b. Rhizoma Gastrodiae Elatae (*Tian Ma*)
    c. Lumbricus (*Di Long*)
    d. Concha Margaritiferae (*Zhen Zhu Mu*)
    e. Periostracum Cicadae (*Chan Tui*)

    Answer: ___

384. Which of the following medicinals drains fire, subdues yang, and brightens the eyes:
    a. Semen Cassiae Torae (*Jue Ming Zi*)
    b. Concha Haliotidis (*Shi Jue Ming*)
    c. Radix Rubrus Paeoniae Lactiflorae (*Chi Shao*)
    d. Spica Prunellae Vulgaris (*Xia Ku Cao*)
    e. Herba Equiseti Hiemalis (*Mu Zei Cao*)

    Answer: ___

385. Which of the following medicinals subdues yang and downbears counterflow:
    a. Magnetitum (*Ci Shi*)
    b. Haemititum (*Dai Zhe Shi*)
    c. Concha Ostreae (*Mu Li*)
    d. Concha Margaritiferae (*Zhen Zhu Mu*)
    e. Dens Draconis (*Long Chi*)

    Answer: ___

386. Which of the following medicinals both levels and soothes the liver:
    a. Rhizoma Cyperi Rotundi (*Xiang Fu*)
    b. Semen Cassiae Torae (*Jue Ming Zi*)
    c. Tuber Curcumae (*Yu Jin*)
    d. Fructus Tribuli Terrestris (*Bai Ji Li*)
    e. Radix Bupleuri (*Chai Hu*)

    Answer: ___

387. Which of the following medicinals levels the liver and brightens the eyes, dispels wind and stops itching:
    a. Fructus Lycii Chinensis (*Gou Qi Zi*)
    b. Concha Haliotidis (*Shi Jue Ming*)
    c. Fructus Tribuli Terrestris (*Bai Ji Li*)
    d. Cortex Radicis Dictamni Dasycarpi (*Bai Xian Pi*)
    e. Herba Menthae Haplocalycis (*Bo He*)

    Answer: ___

388. Which of the following medicinals A) clears the liver and brightens the eyes and B) moistens the intestines and frees the flow of the stools:
    a. Semen Cuscutae Chinensis (*Tu Si Zi*)
    b. Fructus Perillae Frutescentis (*Zi Su Zi*)
    c. Semen Astragali Complanati (*Sha Yuan Zi*)
    d. Semen Plantaginis (*Che Qian Zi*)
    e. Semen Cassiae Torae (*Jue Ming Zi*)

    Answer: ___

389. Which of the following medicinals extinguishes wind, stops tetany, and transforms phlegm:
    a. Radix Polygalae Tenuifoliae (*Yuan Zhi*)
    b. Ramulus Uncariae Cum Uncis (*Gou Teng*)
    c. Bombyx Batryticatus (*Jiang Can*)
    d. Rhizoma Gastrodiae Elatae (*Tian Ma*)
    e. Radix Platycodi Grandiflori (*Jie Geng*)

    Answer: ___

390. Which of the following medicinals clears heat, extinguishes wind, levels panting, frees the flow of the network vessels, and disinhibits urination:
    a. Lumbricus (*Di Long*)
    b. Buthus Martensis (*Quan Xie*)
    c. Scolopendra Subspinipes (*Wu Gong*)
    d. Bombyx Batryticatus (*Jiang Can*)
    e. Agkistrodon Seu Bungarus (*Bai Hua She*)

    Answer: ___

391. Which of the following medicinals A) extinguishes wind and stops tetany, B) resolves fire toxins and scatters nodulations, and C) frees the flow of the network vessels and stops pain:
    a. Bombyx Batryticatus (*Jiang Can*)
    b. Lumbricus (*Di Long*)
    c. Concha Haliotidis (*Shi Jue Ming*)
    d. Buthus Martensis (*Quan Xie*)
    e. Fructus Tribuli Terrestris (*Bai Ji Li*)

    Answer: ___

392. Which of the following pairs of medicinals A) level the liver and subdue yang and B) clear the liver and brighten the eyes:
    a. Spica Prunellae Vulgaris (*Xia Ku Cao*) & Herba Equiseti Hiemalis (*Mu Zei Cao*)
    b. Cornu Antelopis Saiga-tatarici (*Ling Yang Jiao*) & Concha Haliotidis (*Shi Jue Ming*)
    c. Concha Ostreae (*Mu Li*) & Concha Margaritiferae (*Zhen Zhu Mu*)
    d. Concha Haliotidis (*Shi Jue Ming*) & Fructus Tribuli Terrestris (*Bai Ji Li*)
    e. Spica Prunellae Vulgaris (*Xia Ku Cao*) & Semen Cassiae Torae (*Jue Ming Zi*)

    Answer: ___

Orifice-opening Medicinals (*Kai Qiao Yao*)

393. Which of the following medicinals A) open the orifices and arouse the brain and B) treats dead fetus and retention of the placenta:
    a. Styrax Liquidus (*Su He Xiang*)
    b. Cortex Cinnamomi Cassiae (*Rou Gui*)
    c. Radix Achyranthis Bidentatae (*Niu Xi*)
    d. Secretio Moschi Moschiferi (*She Xiang*)
    e. Radix Trichosanthis Kirlowii (*Tian Hua Fen*)

394. Which of the following medicinals is usually used in powder or pill form:
    a. Resina Olibani (*Ru Xiang*)
    b. Rhizoma Cyperi Rotundi (*Xiang Fu*)
    c. Herba Agastachis Seu Pogostemi (*Huo Xiang*)
    d. Fructus Foeniculi Vulgaris (*Xiao Hui Xiang*)
    e. Secretio Moschi Moschiferi (*She Xiang*)

    Answer: ___

395. Borneol (*Bing Pian*)'s functions are to:
    a. Open the orifices and arouse the brain, quicken the blood and dispel stasis
    b. Open the orifices and arouse the brain, clear heat and stop pain
    c. Open the orifices and arouse the brain, eliminate dampness and harmonize the stomach
    d. Open the orifices and arouse the brain, hasten delivery
    e. Open the orifices and arouse the brain, rectify the qi and downbear counterflow

    Answer: ___

396. Which of the following medicinals is used to treat all sorts of sores and tinea, sore throat, mouth sores, and eye diseases:
    a. Cinnabar (*Zhu Sha*)
    b. Secretio Moschi Moschiferi (*She Xiang*)
    c. Borneol (*Bing Pian*)
    d. Realgar (*Xiong Huang*)
    e. Sulphur (*Liu Huang*)

    Answer: ___

397. Rhizoma Acori Graminei (*Shi Chang Pu*)'s functions are to:
    a. Open the orifices and quicken the blood
    b. Open the orifices and clear heat
    c. Open the orifices and transform dampness
    d. Open the orifices and hasten delivery
    e. Open the orifices and disinhibit urination

    Answer: ___

398. Which of the following medicinals treats loss of consciousness due to phlegm dampness confounding the heart orifices with spasms and contractions, vertigo and dizziness, and deafness:
    a. Tuber Curcumae (*Yu Jin*)
    b. Semen Raphani Sativi (*Lai Fu Zi*)
    c. Semen Sinapis Albae (*Bai Jie Zi*)
    d. Agkistrodon Seu Bungarus (*Bai Hua She*)
    e. Rhizoma Acori Graminei (*Shi Chang Pu*)

    Answer: ___

399. Which of the following medicinals A) clears the heart and opens the orifices, B) clears the liver and extinguishes wind, and C) drains heat and resolves fire toxins:
    a. Rhizoma Coptidis Chinensis (*Huang Lian*)
    b. Fructus Gardeniae Jasminoidis (*Shan Zhi Zi*)
    c. Rhizoma Acori Graminei (*Shi Chang Pu*)
    d. Styrax Liquidus (*Su He Xiang*)
    e. Calculus Bovis (*Niu Huang*)

    Answer: ___

Medicinals for External Application (*Wai Fu Yao*)

400. The functions of Alum (*Ku Fan*) when used externally are to:
    a. Resolve toxins and kill worms
    b. Dry dampness and stop itching
    c. Stop bleeding, secure and astringe
    d. All of the above
    e. None of the above

    Answer: ___

401. Realgar (*Xiong Huang*) can be mixed with isopropyl alcohol and applied externally to herpes lesions
    as long as they are:
    a. Dry and scabbing
    b. Open and wet
    c. Red and unruptured
    d. All of the above
    e. None of the above

    Answer: ___

402. Borax (*Peng Sha*) when applied externally:
    a. Dries dampness
    b. Clears heat and resolves toxins
    c. A & B
    d. None of the above

    Answer: ___

403. Sulphur (*Liu Huang*) resolves toxins, kills worms, and stops itching when applied externally, and
    _____ when taken internally:
    a. Dries dampness and transforms phlegm
    b. Clears heat and drains fire
    c. Divides clear from turbid
    d. Supplements lifegate fire and invigorates yang
    e. None of the above

    Answer: ___

404. Fructus Cnidii Monnieri (*She Chuang Zi*):
    a. Dries dampness and kills worms, warms the kidneys and invigorates yang
    b. Dries dampness and kills worms, fortifies the spleen and supplements the qi
    c. Dries dampness and kills worms, moistens the intestines and frees the flow of the stools
    d. Dries dampness and kills worms, moistens the lungs and stops bleeding
    e. Dries dampness and kills worms, secures and astringes, engenders new tissue

    Answer: ___

405. Camphora (*Zhang Nao*):
    a. Dispels wind dampness and kills worms
    b. Opens the orifices and aromatically penetrates turbidity
    c. Quickens the blood and stops pain
    d. A & B
    e. All of the above

    Answer: ___

406. Which of the following medicinals A) brightens the eyes and B) dries dampness and engenders new tissue:
    a. Smithsonitum (*Lu Gan Shi*)
    b. Os Sepiae Seu Sepiellae (*Wu Zei Gu*)
    c. Concha Haliotidis (*Shi Jue Ming*)
    d. Semen Cassiae Torae (*Jue Ming Zi*)
    e. Fructus Schisandrae Chinensis (*Wu Wei Zi*)

    Answer: ___

Miscellaneous Questions on Medicinals

407. Which medicinals free the flow of the network vessels:
   a. Lumbricus (*Di Long*)
   b. Buthus Martensis (*Quan Xie*)
   c. Bombyx Batryticatus (*Jiang Can*)
   d. All of them
   e. None of them

   Answer: ___

408. Which medicinal does not diffuse the lung qi:
   a. Herba Ephedrae (*Ma Huang*)
   b. Radix Platycodi Grandiflori (*Jie Geng*)
   c. Radix Peucedani (*Qian Hu*)
   d. Semen Pruni Armeniacae (*Xing Ren*)
   e. Rhizoma Alismatis (*Ze Xie*)

   Answer: ___

409. Which medicinal does not clear heat from the lungs:
   a. Radix Bupleuri (*Chai Hu*)
   b. Radix Scutellariae Baicalensis (*Huang Qin*)
   c. Cortex Radicis Mori Albi (*Sang Bai Pi*)
   d. Herba Houttuyniae Cordatae Cum Radice (*Yu Xing Cao*)
   e. Flos Lonicerae Japonicae (*Jin Yin Hua*)

   Answer: ___

410. Which medicinal does not moisten the lungs:
   a. Radix Glehniae Littoralis (*Sha Shen*)
   b. Rhizoma Belamcandae (*She Gan*)
   c. Tuber Ophiopogonis Japonici (*Mai Men Dong*)
   d. Tuber Asparagi Cochinensis (*Tian Men Dong*)
   e. Radix Trichosanthis Kirlowii (*Tian Hua Fen*)

   Answer: ___

411. Which medicinal does not downbear the lung qi:
   a. Fructus Perillae Frutescentis (*Zi Su Zi*)
   b. Semen Pruni Armeniacae (*Xing Ren*)
   c. Radix Auklandiae Lappae (*Mu Xiang*)
   d. Cortex Magnoliae Officinalis (*Hou Po*)
   e. Rhizoma Cynanchi Stautonii (*Bai Qian*)

   Answer: ___

412. Which medicinal does not warm the lungs:
    a. dry Rhizoma Zingiberis (*Gan Jiang*)
    b. Herba Asari Cum Radice (*Xi Xin*)
    c. Ramulus Cinnamomi Cassiae (*Gui Zhi*)
    d. Rhizoma Coptidis Chinensis (*Huang Lian*)

    Answer: ___

413. Which medicinal does not transform phlegm:
    a. Rhizoma Pinelliae Ternatae (*Ban Xia*)
    b. Radix Scutellariae Baicalensis (*Huang Qin*)
    c. Rhizoma Arisaematis (*Nan Xing*)
    d. Semen Sinapis Albae (*Bai Jie Zi*)
    e. Pericarpium Citri Reticulatae (*Chen Pi*)

    Answer: ___

414. Which medicinal does not supplement the lung qi:
    a. Radix Polygoni Multiflori (*He Shou Wu*)
    b. Radix Astragali Membranacei (*Huang Qi*)
    c. Radix Panacis Ginseng (*Ren Shen*)
    d. Radix Codonopsitis Pilosulae (*Dang Shen*)

    Answer: ___

415. Which medicinal does not astringe the lungs:
    a. Radix Euryalis Ferocis (*Qian Shi*)
    b. Fructus Schisandrae Chinensis (*Wu Wei Zi*)
    c. Fructus Pruni Mume (*Wu Mei*)
    d. Fructus Terminaliae Chebulae (*He Zi*)
    e. Pericarpium Papaveris Somniferi (*Ying Su Ke*)

    Answer: ___

416. Which medicinal does not supplement heart qi:
    a. Radix Panacis Ginseng (*Ren Shen*)
    b. Radix Salviae Miltiorrhizae (*Dan Shen*)
    c. Radix Codonopsitis Pilosulae (*Dang Shen*)
    d. Radix Pseudostellariae (*Tai Zi Shen*)
    e. Radix Glycyrrhizae (*Gan Cao*)

    Answer: ___

417. Which medicinal does not warm heart yang:
   a. Radix Lateralis Praeparatus Aconiti Carmichaeli (*Fu Zi*)
   b. dry Rhizoma Zingiberis (*Gan Jiang*)
   c. Radix Glehniae Littoralis (*Sha Shen*)
   d. Ramulus Cinnamomi Cassiae (*Gui Zhi*)

   Answer: ___

418. Which medicinal does not supplement heart blood:
   a. Radix Angelicae Sinensis (*Dang Gui*)
   b. cooked Radix Rehmanniae (*Shu Di*)
   c. Radix Platycodi Grandiflori (*Jie Geng*)
   d. Arillus Euphoriae Longanae (*Long Yan Rou*)
   e. Gelatinum Corii Asini (*E Jiao*)

   Answer: ___

419. Which medicinal does not clear heart fire:
   a. Rhizoma Coptidis Chinensis (*Huang Lian*)
   b. Rhizoma Cyperi Rotundi (*Xiang Fu*)
   c. uncooked Radix Rehmanniae (*Sheng Di*)
   d. Folium Lophatheri Gracilis (*Dan Zhu Ye*)
   e. Caulis Akebiae (*Mu Tong*)

   Answer: ___

420. Which medicinal does not nourish the heart and quiet the spirit:
   a. Rhizoma Coptidis Chinensis (*Huang Lian*)
   b. Semen Biotae Orientalis (*Bai Zi Ren*)
   c. Semen Zizyphi Spinosae (*Suan Zao Ren*)
   d. Fructus Zizyphi Jujubae (*Da Zao*)
   e. Caulis Polygoni Multiflori (*Ye Jiao Teng*)

   Answer: ___

421. Which medicinal does not open the orifices:
   a. Secretio Moschi Moschiferi (*She Xiang*)
   b. Borneolum (*Bing Pian*)
   c. Styrax Liquidus (*Su He Xiang*)
   d. Rhizoma Acori Graminei (*Shi Chang Pu*)
   e. Radix Salviae Miltiorrhizae (*Dan Shen*)

   Answer: ___

422. Which medicinal does not quicken the blood:
    a. Semen Pruni Persicae (*Tao Ren*)
    b. Radix Bupleuri (*Chai Hu*)
    c. Radix Ligustici Wallichii (*Chuan Xiong*)
    d. Flos Carthami Tinctorii (*Hong Hua*)
    e. Radix Angelicae Sinensis (*Dang Gui*)

    Answer: ___

423. Which medicinal does not supplement the spleen qi:
    a. Radix Panacis Ginseng (*Ren Shen*)
    b. Radix Scutellariae Baicalensis (*Huang Qin*)
    c. Rhizoma Atractylodis Macrocephalae (*Bai Zhu*)
    d. Radix Dioscoreae Oppositae (*Shan Yao*)
    e. Radix Astragali Membranacei (*Huang Qi*)

    Answer: ___

424. Which medicinal does not warm spleen yang:
    a. Semen Raphani Sativi (*Lai Fu Zi*)
    b. dry Rhizoma Zingiberis (*Gan Jiang*)
    c. Cortex Cinnamomi Cassiae (*Rou Gui*)
    d. Ramulus Cinnamomi Cassiae (*Gui Zhi*)
    e. Radix Lateralis Praeparatus Aconiti Carmichaeli (*Fu Zi*)

    Answer: ___

425. Which medicinal does not upbear the central qi:
    a. Radix Astragali Membranacei (*Huang Qi*)
    b. Rhizoma Cimicifugae (*Sheng Ma*)
    c. Pericarpium Citri Reticulatae (*Chen Pi*)
    d. Radix Puerariae (*Ge Gen*)
    e. Radix Bupleuri (*Chai Hu*)

    Answer: ___

426. Which medicinal does not eliminate dampness:
    a. Rhizoma Atractylodis (*Cang Zhu*)
    b. Herba Eupatorii (*Pei Lan*)
    c. Cortex Magnoliae Officinalis (*Hou Po*)
    d. Tuber Ophiopogonis Japonici (*Mai Men Dong*)
    e. Fructus Cardamomi (*Bai Dou Kou*)

    Answer: ___

427. Which medicinal does not regulate the spleen qi:
    a. Radix Angelicae Sinensis (*Dang Gui*)
    b. Radix Auklandiae Lappae (*Mu Xiang*)
    c. Fructus Citri Aurantii (*Zhi Ke*)
    d. Caulis Perillae Frutescentis (*Su Gen*)
    e. Fructus Amomi (*Sha Ren*)

    Answer: ___

428. Which medicinal does not clear stomach heat:
    a. Rhizoma Coptidis Chinensis (*Huang Lian*)
    b. Gypsum Fibrosum (*Shi Gao*)
    c. uncooked Rhizoma Zingiberis (*Sheng Jiang*)
    d. Radix Et Rhizoma Rhei (*Da Huang*)
    e. Rhizoma Phragmitis Communis (*Lu Gen*)

    Answer: ___

429. Which medicinal does not nourish stomach yin:
    a. Rhizoma Cyperi Rotundi (*Xiang Fu*)
    b. Herba Dendrobii (*Shi Hu*)
    c. Tuber Ophiopogonis Japonici (*Mai Men Dong*)
    d. Radix Glehniae Littoralis (*Sha Shen*)
    e. Rhizoma Polygonati Odorati (*Yu Zhu*)

    Answer: ___

430. Which medicinal does not downbear the stomach qi:
    a. uncooked Rhizoma Zingiberis (*Sheng Jiang*)
    b. Radix Puerariae (*Ge Gen*)
    c. Flos Caryophylli (*Ding Xiang*)
    d. Rhizoma Pinelliae Ternatae (*Ban Xia*)
    e. Fructus Evodiae Rutecarpae (*Wu Zhu Yu*)

    Answer: ___

431. Which medicinal does not disperse food accumulations:
    a. Fructus Crataegi (*Shan Zha*)
    b. Massa Medica Fermentata (*Shen Qu*)
    c. Fructus Germinatus Hordei Vulgaris (*Mai Ya*)
    d. Endothelium Corneum Gigeriae Galli (*Ji Nei Jin*)
    e. Rhizoma Alismatis (*Ze Xie*)

    Answer: ___

432. Which medicinal does not moisten the intestines and free the flow of the stools:
    a. Semen Cannabis Sativae (*Huo Ma Ren*)
    b. Semen Pruni (*Yu Li Ren*)
    c. Tuber Ophiopogonis Japonici (*Mai Men Dong*)
    d. Radix Angelicae Sinensis (*Dang Gui*)
    e. Herba Cistanchis Deserticolae (*Rou Cong Rong*)

    Answer: ___

433. Which medicinal does not clear damp heat from the large intestine:
    a. Rhizoma Coptidis Chinensis (*Huang Lian*)
    b. Radix Pulsatillae Chinese (*Bai Tou Weng*)
    c. Cortex Fraxini (*Qin Pi*)
    d. Fructus Amomi (*Sha Ren*)
    e. Cortex Phellodendri (*Huang Bai*)

    Answer: ___

434. Which medicinal does not astringe the intestines and stop diarrhea:
    a. Fructus Pruni Mume (*Wu Mei*)
    b. Fructus Schisandrae Chinensis (*Wu Wei Zi*)
    c. Semen Myristicae Fragrantis (*Rou Dou Kou*)
    d. Fructus Terminaliae Chebulae (*He Zi*)
    e. Rhizoma Coptidis Chinensis (*Huang Lian*)

    Answer: ___

435. Which medicinal does not clear liver heat:
    a. Rhizoma Cyperi Rotundi (*Xiang Fu*)
    b. Radix Gentianae Scabrae (*Long Dan Cao*)
    c. Fructus Gardeniae Jasminoidis (*Shan Zhi Zi*)
    d. Radix Scutellariae Baicalensis (*Huang Qin*)
    e. Flos Chrysanthemi Morifolii (*Ju Hua*)

    Answer: ___

436. Which medicinal does not subdue ascendant liver yang hyperactivity:
    a. Concha Haliotidis (*Shi Jue Ming*)
    b. Rhizoma Coptidis Chinensis (*Huang Lian*)
    c. Concha Ostreae (*Mu Li*)
    d. Plastrum Testudinis (*Gui Ban*)
    e. Carapax Amydae Sinensis (*Bei Jia*)

    Answer: ___

437. Which medicinal does not extinguish liver wind:
    a. Cornu Antelopis Saiga-tatarici (*Ling Yang Jiao*)
    b. Rhizoma Pinelliae Ternatae (*Ban Xia*)
    c. Rhizoma Gastrodiae Elatae (*Tian Ma*)
    d. Ramulus Uncariae Cum Uncis (*Gou Teng*)
    e. Fructus Tribuli Terrestris (*Bai Ji Li*)

    Answer: ___

438. Which medicinal does not nourish liver yin:
    a. cooked Radix Rehmanniae (*Shu Di*)
    b. Fructus Lycii Chinensis (*Gou Qi Zi*)
    c. Radix Polygoni Multiflori (*He Shou Wu*)
    d. Radix Bupleuri (*Chai Hu*)
    e. Radix Albus Paeoniae Lactiflorae (*Bai Shao*)

    Answer: ___

439. Which medicinal does not quicken the blood:
    a. Herba Leonuri Heterophylli (*Yi Mu Cao*)
    b. Radix Ligustici Wallichii (*Chuan Xiong*)
    c. Radix Auklandiae Lappae (*Mu Xiang*)
    d. Flos Carthami Tinctorii (*Hong Hua*)
    d. Semen Pruni Persicae (*Tao Ren*)

    Answer: ___

440. Which medicinal does not clear heat from the gallbladder:
    a. Radix Gentianae Scabrae (*Long Dan Cao*)
    b. Radix Linderae Strychnifoliae (*Wu Yao*)
    c. Radix Scutellariae Baicalensis (*Huang Qin*)
    d. Herba Artemisiae Capillaris (*Yin Chen Hao*)
    e. Fructus Gardeniae Jasminoidis (*Shan Zhi Zi*)

    Answer: ___

441. Which medicinal does not supplement the kidneys and invigorate yang:
    a. Rhizoma Curculiginis Orchioidis (*Xian Mao*)
    b. Herba Epimedii (*Xian Ling Pi*)
    c. Herba Cistanchis Deserticolae (*Rou Cong Rong*)
    d. Herba Cynomorii Songarici (*Suo Yang*)
    e. Fructus Meliae Toosendan (*Chuan Lian Zi*)

    Answer: ___

442. Which medicinal does not strengthen the sinews and strengthen the bones:
    a. Cortex Eucommiae Ulmoidis (*Du Zhong*)
    b. Radix Dipsaci (*Xu Duan*)
    c. Radix Dioscoreae Oppositae (*Shan Yao*)
    d. Ramulus Loranthi Seu Visci (*Sang Ji Sheng*)
    e. Cortex Radicis Acanthopanacis Gracilistyli (*Wu Jia Pi*)

    Answer: ___

443. Which medicinal does not supplement the kidneys and promote the kidneys' grasping or absorbing of qi:
    a. Semen Cuscutae Chinensis (*Tu Si Zi*)
    b. Semen Juglandis Regiae (*Hu Tao Ren*)
    c. Gecko (*Ge Jie*)
    d. Fructus Schisandrae Chinensis (*Wu Wei Zi*)
    e. Cordyceps (*Dong Chong Xia Cao*)

    Answer: ___

444. Which medicinal does not enrich kidney yin:
    a. Cortex Radicis Moutan (*Dan Pi*)
    b. cooked Radix Rehmanniae (*Shu Di*)
    c. Fructus Ligustri Lucidi (*Nu Zhen Zi*)
    d. Herba Ecliptae Prostratae (*Han Lian Cao*)
    e. Plastrum Testudinis (*Gui Ban*)

    Answer: ___

445. Which medicinal does not clear vacuity heat:
    a. Rhizoma Anemarrhenae Aspheloidis (*Zhi Mu*)
    b. Cortex Phellodendri (*Huang Bai*)
    c. Radix Pulsatillae Chinensis (*Bai Tou Weng*)
    d. Cortex Radicis Moutan (*Dan Pi*)
    e. Radix Gentianae Macrophyllae (*Qin Jiao*)

    Answer: ___

446. Which medicinal does not disinhibit urination:
    a. Sclerotium Poriae Cocos (*Fu Ling*)
    b. Pericarpium Citri Reticulatae (*Chen Pi*)
    c. Sclerotium Polypori Umbellati (*Zhu Ling*)
    d. Rhizoma Alismatis (*Ze Xie*)
    e. Semen Plantaginis (*Che Qian Zi*)

    Answer: ___

447. Which medicinal does not quicken the network vessels:
    a. Resina Olibani (*Ru Xiang*)
    b. Resina Myrrhae (*Mo Yao*)
    c. Radix Polygalae Tenuifoliae (*Yuan Zhi*)
    d. Buthus Martensis (*Quan Xie*)
    e. Fascicularis Vascularis Luffae Cylindricae (*Xi Gua Luo*)

    Answer: ___

448. Which medicinal does not open the orifice of the nose:
    a. Herba Menthae Haplocalycis (*Bo He*)
    b. Fructus Schisandrae Chinensis (*Wu Wei Zi*)
    c. Radix Angelicae Dahuricae (*Bai Zhi*)
    d. Fructus Xanthii Sibirici (*Cang Er Zi*)
    e. Flos Magnoliae Liliflorae (*Xin Yi Hua*)

    Answer: ___

449. Which medicinal does not secure the essence and stop leakage:
    a. Semen Cuscutae Chinensis (*Tu Si Zi*)
    b. Semen Euryalis Ferocis (*Qian Shi*)
    c. Ootheca Mantidis (*Sang Piao Xiao*)
    d. Fructus Corni Officinalis (*Shan Zhu Yu*)
    e. Fructus Mori Albi (*Sang Shen*)

    Answer: ___

450. Which medicinal does not rectify the qi:
    a. Radix Albus Paeoniae Lactiflorae (*Bai Shao*)
    b. Radix Bupleuri (*Chai Hu*)
    c. Rhizoma Cyperi Rotundi (*Xiang Fu*)
    d. Fructus Meliae Toosendan (*Chuan Lian Zi*)
    e. Radix Auklandiae Lappae (*Mu Xiang*)

    Answer: ___

451. For water swelling due to spleen and kidney yang vacuity, use:
    a. dry Rhizoma Zingiberis (*Gan Jiang*) & Radix Glycyrrhizae (*Gan Cao*)
    b. Radix Panacis Ginseng (*Ren Shen*) & Radix Glycyrrhizae (*Gan Cao*)
    c. Cortex Cinnamomi Cassiae (*Rou Gui*) & Fructus Corni Officinalis (*Shan Zhu Yu*)
    d. Radix Panacis Ginseng (*Ren Shen*) & Rhizoma Atractylodis Macrocephalae (*Bai Zhu*)
    e. Radix Lateralis Praeparatus Aconiti Carmichaeli (*Fu Zi*) & Sclerotium Poriae Cocos (*Fu Ling*)

    Answer: ___

452. Flos Chrysanthemi Morifolii (*Ju Hua*), Radix Gentianae Scabrae (*Long Dan Cao*), and Cortex Radicis Moutan (*Dan Pi*) all:
    a. Dispel wind and clear heat
    b. Clear heat, resolve toxins, and cool the blood
    c. Clear and drain liver and gallbladder damp heat
    d. Level the liver and extinguish wind
    e. None of the above

    Answer: ___

453. Herba Agastachis Seu Pogostemi (*Huo Xiang*), Herba Elsholtziae (*Xiang Ru*), and Herba Eupatorii Fortunei (*Pei Lan*) all can be used for:
    a. External contraction of wind cold
    b. External contraction of summerheat dampness
    c. Damp turbidity obstructing the middle
    d. Water swelling and strangury
    e. Nausea and vomiting

    Answer: ___

454. Cortex Eucommiae Ulmoidis (*Du Zhong*) and Ramulus Loranthi Seu Visci (*Sang Ji Sheng*) both:
    a. Supplement the liver and kidneys and disinhibit urination
    b. Quicken the blood and supplement the liver and kidneys
    c. Quicken the blood and quiet the fetus
    d. Quiet the fetus and supplement the liver and kidneys
    e. Disinhibit urination and quiet the fetus

    Answer: ___

455. Rhizoma Coptidis Chinensis (*Huang Lian*), uncooked Rhizoma Zingiberis (*Sheng Jiang*), and Fructus Evodiae Rutecarpae (*Wu Zhu Yu*) all:
    a. Clear heat
    b. Dispel cold
    c. Stop vomiting
    d. Stop pain
    e. Stop diarrhea

    Answer: ___

456. To treat rib-side pain due to liver depression qi stagnation, Rhizoma Cyperi Rotundi (*Xiang Fu*) should be combined with:
    a. Radix Auklandiae Lappae (*Mu Xiang*) & Radix Linderae Strychnifoliae (*Wu Yao*)
    b. Radix Bupleuri (*Chai Hu*) & Radix Albus Paeoniae Lactiflorae (*Bai Shao*)
    c. Fructus Foeniculi Vulgaris (*Xiao Hui Xiang*) & Radix Linderae Strychnifoliae (*Wu Yao*)
    d. Rhizoma Alpiniae Officinari (*Gao Liang Jiang*) & dry Rhizoma Zingiberis (*Gan Jiang*)
    e. None of the above

    Answer: ___

457. To treat dysentery with abdominal pain, tenesmus, and pus and blood in the stools (*i.e.*, red and white dysentery), the best combination is:
    a. Rhizoma Coptidis Chinensis (*Huang Lian*) & Radix Auklandiae Lappae (*Mu Xiang*)
    b. Rhizoma Coptidis Chinensis (*Huang Lian*) & Radix Puerariae (*Ge Gen*)
    c. Rhizoma Coptidis Chinensis (*Huang Lian*) & Cortex Fraxini (*Qin Pi*)
    d. Rhizoma Coptidis Chinensis (*Huang Lian*) & Fructus Gardeniae Jasminoidis (*Shan Zhi Zi*)
    e. Rhizoma Coptidis Chinensis (*Huang Lian*) & Semen Arecae Catechu (*Bing Lang*)

    Answer: ___

458. Which is the best pair for treating vexation and insomnia due to heart fire hyperactivity:
    a. Rhizoma Coptidis Chinensis (*Huang Lian*) & Gelatinum Corii Asini (*E Jiao*)
    b. Os Draconis (*Long Gu*) & Concha Ostreae (*Mu Li*)
    c. Semen Zizyphi Spinosae (*Suan Zao Ren*) & Semen Biotae Orientalis (*Bai Zi Ren*)
    d. Cinnabar (*Zhu Sha*) & Magnetitum (*Ci Shi*)
    e. Caulis Polygoni Multiflori (*Ye Jiao Teng*) & Cortex Albizziae Julibrissinis (*He Huan Pi*)

    Answer: ___

459. Which is the best pair for treating poor appetite, loose stools, and loss of strength in the four extremities due to spleen qi vacuity:
    a. Rhizoma Atractylodis Macrocephalae (*Bai Zhu*) & Sclerotium Poriae Cocos (*Fu Ling*)
    b. Fructus Terminaliae Chebulae (*He Zi*) & Semen Myristicae Fragrantis (*Rou Dou Kou*)
    c. Radix Auklandiae Lappae (*Mu Xiang*) & Fructus Chaenomelis Lagenariae (*Mu Gua*)
    d. Radix Angelicae Sinensis (*Dang Gui*) & Caulis Milletiae Seu Spatholobi (*Ji Xue Teng*)
    e. Radix Astragali Membranacei (*Huang Qi*) & Radix Angelicae Sinensis (*Dang Gui*)

    Answer: ___

460. Radix Ligustici Wallichii (*Chuan Xiong*) should be combined with _____ for the treatment of rib-side pain due to qi stagnation and blood stasis:
    a. Herba Leonuri Heterophylli (*Yi Mu Cao*) & Semen Pruni Persicae (*Tao Ren*)
    b. Radix Rubrus Paeoniae Lactiflorae (*Chi Shao*) & Cortex Radicis Moutan (*Dan Pi*)
    c. Radix Bupleuri (*Chai Hu*) & Rhizoma Cyperi Rotundi (*Xiang Fu*)
    d. Radix Achyranthis Bidentatae (*Niu Xi*) & Plastrum Testudinis (*Gui Ban*)
    e. Carapax Amydae Sinensis (*Bei Jia*) & Succinum (*Hu Po*)

    Answer: ___

461. For severe qi vacuity and yang desertion with chilled extremities, profuse sweating, weak breathing, and a faint (*wei*) pulse, use:
    a. Radix Lateralis Praeparatus Aconiti Carmichaeli (*Fu Zi*) & Radix Astragali Membranacei (*Huang Qi*)
    b. Radix Lateralis Praeparatus Aconiti Carmichaeli (*Fu Zi*) & Radix Panacis Ginseng (*Ren Shen*)
    c. Rhizoma Atractylodis Macrocephalae (*Bai Zhu*) & Radix Lateralis Praeparatus Aconiti Carmichaeli (*Fu Zi*)
    d. Radix Lateralis Praeparatus Aconiti Carmichaeli (*Fu Zi*) & dry Rhizoma Zingiberis (*Gan Jiang*)
    e. Radix Lateralis Praeparatus Aconiti Carmichaeli (*Fu Zi*) & Cortex Cinnamomi Cassiae (*Rou Gui*)

    Answer: ___

462. Magnetitum (*Ci Shi*), Concha Ostreae (*Mu Li*), and Os Draconis (*Long Gu*) should all be:
    a. Decocted first
    b. Decocted after
    c. Dissolved in the strained decoction
    d. Steeped
    e. None of the above

    Answer: ___

463. Radix Stephaniae Tetrandrae (*Fang Ji*) and Radix Ledebouriellae Divaricatae (*Fang Feng*) both:
    a. Disinhibit urination and disperse swelling
    b. Dispel wind and resolve the exterior
    c. Disinhibit urination and free the flow of strangury
    d. Dispel wind and eliminate dampness
    e. Eliminate dampness and recede or abate jaundice

    Answer: ___

464. Which pair of medicinals can transform phlegm and stop vomiting:
    a. Radix Platycodi Grandiflori (*Jie Geng*) & Flos Inulae (*Xuan Fu Hua*)
    b. Flos Inulae (*Xuan Fu Hua*) & Rhizoma Pinelliae Ternatae (*Ban Xia*)
    c. Rhizoma Pinelliae Ternatae (*Ban Xia*) & Rhizoma Phragmitis Communis (*Lu Gen*)
    d. Rhizoma Phragmitis Communis (*Lu Gen*) & Caulis Bambusae In Taeniis (*Zhu Ru*)
    e. Caulis Bambusae In Taeniis (*Zhu Ru*) & Radix Platycodi Grandiflori (*Jie Geng*)

    Answer: ___

465. Cinnabar (*Zhu Sha*), Caulis Akebiae (*Mu Tong*), Folium Lophatheri Gracilis (*Dan Zhu Ye*), and Tuber Curcumae (*Yu Jin*) all:
    a. Clear heart fire
    b. Clear heat and resolve toxins
    c. Quicken the blood and dispel stasis
    d. Clear liver fire
    e. None of the above

    Answer: ___

466. Os Draconis (*Long Gu*) and Concha Ostreae (*Mu Li*) both:
    a. Nourish the heart and quiet the spirit
    b. Astringe and secure, restrain and contain
    c. Soften the hard and dispel stasis
    d. Enrich yin and subdue yang
    e. All of the above

    Answer: ___

467. Radix Angelicae Sinensis (*Dang Gui*), Semen Trichosanthis Kirlowii (*Gua Lou Ren*), Herba Cistanchis Deserticolae (*Rou Cong Rong*), and Radix Polygoni Multiflori (*He Shou Wu*) all:
   a. Moisten the lungs and stop cough
   b. Supplement the kidneys and invigorate yang
   c. Nourish the blood and regulate menstruation
   d. Moisten the intestines and free the flow of the stools
   e. Dispel wind and stop itching

   Answer: ___

468. Semen Cassiae Torae (*Jue Ming Zi*), Spica Prunellae Vulgaris (*Xia Ku Cao*), Folium Mori Albi (*Sang Ye*), and Cortex Fraxini (*Qin Pi*) all treat:
   a. Liver fire red eyes
   b. Damp heat dysentery
   c. Intestinal dryness constipation
   d. Exterior wind heat patterns
   e. None of the above

   Answer: ___

469. Flos Inulae (*Xuan Fu Hua*) and Haemititum (*Dai Zhe Shi*) both:
   a. Transform phlegm
   b. Subdue yang
   c. Downbear counterflow
   d. Level the liver
   e. All of the above

   Answer: ___

470. Radix Stemonae (*Bai Bu*) and Bulbus Lilii (*Bai He*) both:
   a. Moisten the lungs and stop cough
   b. Kill worms
   c. Clear heat and quiet the spirit
   d. Secure the lungs and stop cough
   e. Nourish the heart and quiet the spirit

   Answer: ___

471. Rhizoma Arisaematis (*Tian Nan Xing*) and Periostracum Cicadae (*Chan Tui*) both:
   a. Dry dampness and transform phlegm
   b. Promote sweating and resolve the exterior
   c. Out-thrust rashes
   d. Brighten the eyes
   e. Dispel wind and stop tetany

   Answer: ___

472. Feces Trogopterori Seu Pteromi (*Wu Ling Zhi*) and Pollen Typhae (*Pu Huang*) both:
    a. Quicken the blood and stop bleeding
    b. Stop bleeding and disinhibit urination
    c. Quicken and cool the blood
    d. Stop bleeding and resolve toxins
    e. None of the above

    Answer: ___

473. Rhizoma Imperatae Cylindricae (*Bai Mao Gen*), Rhizoma Guanchong (*Guan Zhong*), Radix Sanguisorbae (*Di Yu*), and Herba Ecliptae Prostratae (*Han Lian Cao*) all:
    a. Clear heat and disinhibit urination
    b. Supplement the liver and kidneys
    c. Cool the blood and stop bleeding
    d. Kill worms
    e. None of the above

    Answer: ___

474. Sclerotium Poriae Cocos (*Fu Ling*), Rhizoma Atractylodis Macrocephalae (*Bai Zhu*), Semen Coicis Lachryma-jobi (*Yi Yi Ren*), and Radix Dioscoreae Oppositae (*Shan Yao*) all treat:
    a. Spleen vacuity diarrhea
    b. Seminal emission and polyuria
    c. Heart palpitations and insomnia
    d. Exterior vacuity spontaneous perspiration
    e. None of the above

    Answer: ___

475. Flos Caryophylli (*Ding Xiang*), Fructus Cnidii Monnieri (*She Chuang Zi*), Radix Lateralis Praeparatus Aconiti Carmichaeli *(Fu Zi)*, and Fructus Psoraleae Corylifoliae (*Bu Gu Zhi*) all:
    a. Moisten the intestines and free the flow of the stools
    b. Warm the middle and stop vomiting
    c. Warm the kidneys and promote their grasping or absorption of the qi
    d. Supplement the kidneys and invigorate yang
    e. None of the above

    Answer: ___

476. Radix Glycyrrhizae (*Gan Cao*), Rhizoma Cimicifugae (*Sheng Ma*), Rhizoma Guanchong (*Guan Zhong*), and Cornu Antelopis Saiga-tatarici (*Ling Yang Jiao*) all:
    a. Supplement the spleen qi
    b. Clear heat and resolve toxins
    c. Cool the blood and stop bleeding
    d. Level the liver and extinguish wind
    e. None of the above

    Answer: ___

477. Semen Plantaginis (*Che Qian Zi*) and Semen Cassiae Torae (*Jue Ming Zi*) both:
  a. Clear the liver and brighten the eyes
  b. Moisten the intestines and free the flow of the stools
  c. Seep dampness and stop diarrhea
  d. Disinhibit urination and free the flow of strangury
  e. Transform phlegm and stop coughing

  Answer: ___

478. Herba Houttuyniae Cordatae Cum Radice (*Yu Xing Cao*), Rhizoma Phragmitis Communis (*Lu Gen*), Semen Coicis Lachryma-jobi (*Yi Yi Ren*), and Radix Platycodi Grandiflori (*Jie Geng*) all treat:
  a. Sores due to heat toxins
  b. Lung abscess causing chest pain
  c. Damp heat dysentery
  d. Red, painful eyes due to liver fire
  e. None of the above

  Answer: ___

479. Semen Pharbiditis (*Qian Niu Zi*), Radix Stemonae (*Bai Bu*), Fructus Meliae Toosendan (*Chuan Lian Zi*), and Pericarpium Punicae Granati (*Shi Liu Pi*) all:
  a. Drastically precipitate
  b. Kill worms
  c. Rectify the qi and stop pain
  d. Stop diarrhea
  e. None of the above

  Answer: ___

480. Radix Gentianae Macrophyllae (*Qin Jiao*), Cortex Phellodendri (*Huang Bai*), Cortex Radicis Moutan (*Dan Pi*), and Carapax Amydae Sinensis (*Bei Jia*) all:
  a. Treat wind damp impediment pain
  b. Clear and eliminate dampness and heat and stop abnormal vaginal discharge
  c. Cool the blood and stop bleeding
  d. Clear vacuity heat
  e. None of the above

  Answer: ___

481. Radix Scrophulariae Ningpoensis (*Xuan Shen*), Concha Ostreae (*Mu Li*), Bulbus Fritillariae Thunbergii (*Zhe Bei Mu*), and Bombyx Batryticatus (*Jiang Can*) all:
  a. Transform phlegm and stop coughing
  b. Level the liver and subdue yang
  c. Clear heat and disinhibit the throat
  d. Scatter nodulations
  e. None of the above

  Answer: ___

482. Cortex Radicis Moutan (*Dan Pi*), Herba Patriniae Heterophyllae Cum Radice (*Bai Jiang Cao*), Radix Et Rhizoma Rhei (*Da Huang*), and Semen Coicis Lachryma-jobi (*Yi Yi Ren*) all treat:
    a. Intestinal abscess
    b. Enduring vacuity heat
    c. Damp heat jaundice
    d. Heat accumulation constipation
    e. None of the above

    Answer: ___

483. Flos Chrysanthemi Morifolii (*Ju Hua*), Magnetitum (*Ci Shi*), Radix Albus Paeoniae Lactiflorae (*Bai Shao*), and Haemititum (*Dai Zhe Shi*) all:
    a. Clear the liver and brighten the eyes
    b. Level the liver and subdue yang
    c. Clear heat and resolve toxins
    d. Extinguish wind and stop tetany
    e. None of the above

    Answer: ___

484. Rhizoma Cyperi Rotundi (*Xiang Fu*), Pericarpium Citri Reticulatae Viride (*Qing Pi*), Fructus Tribuli Terrestris (*Bai Ji Li*), and Radix Bupleuri (*Chai Hu*) all:
    a. Dispel wind and brighten the eyes
    b. Level the liver and subdue yang
    c. Course the liver and rectify the qi
    d. Dispel wind and stop itching
    e. Break the qi

    Answer: ___

485. Fructus Perillae Frutescentis (*Zi Su Zi*) and Semen Juglandis Regiae (*Hu Tao Ren*) both level panting and:
    a. Supplement the kidneys
    b. Moisten the intestines
    c. Stop pain
    d. Clear heat
    e. Disinhibit urination

    Answer: ___

Formulas (*Fang Ji*)

486. Which is the better formula for a wind heat exterior pattern with cough:
    a. *Sang Ju Yin* (Morus & Chrysanthemum Drink)
    b. *Yin Qiao San* (Lonicera & Forsythia Powder)

    Answer: ___

487. Which is the better formula for a wind cold pattern complicated by vacuity:
    a. *Ma Huang Tang* (Ephedra Decoction)
    b. *Gui Zhi Tang* (Cinnamon Twig Decoction)

    Answer: ___

488. Which is the better formula for a wind cold exterior pattern complicated by phlegm rheum:
    a. *Da Qing Long Tang* (Major Blue-green Dragon Decoction)
    b. *Xiao Qing Long Tang* (Minor Blue-green Dragon Decoction)

    Answer: ___

489. Which is the best formula for *yang ming* heat with concomitant yin vacuity:
    a. *Da Cheng Qi Tang* (Major Order the Qi Decoction)
    b. *Xiao Cheng Qi Tang* (Minor Order the Qi Decoction)
    c. *Zeng Ye Cheng Qi Tang* (Increase Fluids & Order the Qi Decoction)

    Answer: ___

490. Which is the best formula for blood division heat:
    a. *Bai Hu Tang* (White Tiger Decoction)
    b. *Xi Jiao Di Huang Tang* (Rhinoceros Horn & Rehmannia Decoction)
    c. *Qing Wei Tang* (Clear the Stomach Decoction)
    d. *Yu Nu Jian* (Jade Maiden Decoction)
    e. *Qing Ying Tang* (Clear the Constructive Decoction)

    Answer: ___

491. Which is the best formula for blood vacuity and stagnation of cold in the channels and network vessels:
    a. *Li Zhong Wan* (Rectify the Center Pills)
    b. *Xiao Jian Zhong Tang* (Minor Fortify the Center Decoction)
    c. *Zhen Wu Tang* (True Warrior Decoction)
    d. *Xiao Chai Hu Tang* (Minor Bupleurum Decoction)
    e. *Dang Gui Si Ni Tang* (Dang Gui Four Counterflows Decoction)

    Answer: ___

492. Which is the best formula for supplementing kidney yin:
   a. *Liu Wei Di Huang Wan* (Six Flavors Rehmannia Pills)
   b. *Ba Wei Di Huang Wan* (Eight Flavors Rehmannia Pills), a.k.a. *Shen Qi Wan* (Kidney Qi Pills)
   c. *Zhi Bai Di Huang Wan* (Anemarrhena & Phellodendron Rehmannia Pills)
   d. *Si Wu Tang* (Four Materials Decoction)
   e. *Si Jun Zi Tang* (Four Gentlemen Decoction)

   Answer: ___

493. Which is the best formula for supplementing a spleen vacuity with concomitant stomach and intestine qi stagnation:
   a. *Si Jun Zi Tang* (Four Gentlemen Decoction)
   b. *Si Wu Tang* (Four Materials Decoction)
   c. *Xiang Sha Liu Jun Zi Tang* (Auklandia & Amomum Six Gentlemen Decoction)
   d. *Bu Zhong Yi Qi Tang* (Supplement the Center & Boost the Qi Decoction)
   e. *Shen Ling Bai Zhu San* (Ginseng, Poria & Atractylodes Powder)

   Answer: ___

494. Which is the best formula for supplementing both kidney yin and yang:
   a. *Zhen Wu Tang* (True Warrior Decoction)
   b. *Shi Quan Da Bu Tang* (Ten [Ingredients] Completely & Greatly Supplementing Decoction)
   c. *Shen Qi Wan* (Kidney Qi Pills)
   d. *Liu Wei Di Huang Wan* (Six Flavors Rehmannia Pills)
   e. *Zhi Bai Di Huang Wan* (Anemarrhena & Phellodendron Rehmannia Pills)

   Answer: ___

495. Which is the best formula for stopping urinary tract bleeding due to heart heat:
   a. *Huai Hua San* (Immature Sophora Powder)
   b. *Dao Chi San* (Abduct the Red Powder)
   c. *Huang Tu Tang* (Yellow Earth Decoction)
   d. *Dan Zhi Xiao Yao San* (Moutan & Gardenia Rambling Powder)
   e. *Xiao Chai Hu Tang* (Minor Bupleurum Decoction)

   Answer: ___

496. Which is not an ingredient in *Er Chen Tang* (Two Aged [Ingredients] Decoction):
   a. Sclerotium Poriae Cocos (*Fu Ling*)
   b. Radix Glycyrrhizae (*Gan Cao*)
   c. Rhizoma Pinelliae Ternatae (*Ban Xia*)
   d. Pericarpium Citri Reticulatae (*Chen Pi*)
   e. Semen Pruni Armeniacae (*Xing Ren*)

   Answer: ___

497. Which is not an ingredient in *Si Jun Zi Tang* (Four Gentlemen Decoction):
    a. Radix Panacis Ginseng (*Ren Shen*)
    b. Radix Glycyrrhizae (*Gan Cao*)
    c. Rhizoma Atractylodis Macrocephalae (*Bai Zhu*)
    d. Pericarpium Citri Reticulatae (*Chen Pi*)
    e. Sclerotium Poriae Cocos (*Fu Ling*)

    Answer: ___

498. Which is not an ingredient in *Si Wu Tang* (Four Materials Decoction):
    a. cooked Radix Rehmanniae (*Shu Di*)
    b. Radix Albus Paeoniae Lactiflorae (*Bai Shao*)
    c. Fructus Lycii Chinensis (*Gou Qi Zi*)
    d. Radix Angelicae Sinensis (*Dang Gui*)
    e. Radix Ligustici Wallichii (*Chuan Xiong*)

    Answer: ___

499. Which is not an ingredient in *Xiao Chai Hu Tang* (Minor Bupleurum Decoction):
    a. Radix Bupleuri (*Chai Hu*)
    b. Rhizoma Coptidis Chinensis (*Huang Lian*)
    c. Radix Scutellariae Baicalensis (*Huang Qin*)
    d. Rhizoma Pinelliae Ternatae (*Ban Xia*)
    e. Fructus Zizyphi Jujubae (*Da Zao*)

    Answer: ___

500. Which is not an ingredient in *Xiao Yao San* (Rambling Powder):
    a. Herba Mentha Haplocalycis (*Bo He*)
    b. uncooked Rhizoma Zingiberis (*Sheng Jiang*)
    c. Radix Bupleuri (*Chai Hu*)
    d. Radix Codonopsitis Pilosulae (*Dang Shen*)
    e. Sclerotium Poriae Cocos (*Fu Ling*)

    Answer: ___

501. Which is not an ingredient in *Er Xian Tang* (Two Immortals Decoction):
    a. Rhizoma Coptidis Chinensis (*Huang Lian*)
    b. Rhizoma Anemarrhenae Aspheloidis (*Zhi Mu*)
    c. Cortex Phellodendri (*Huang Bai*)
    d. Radix Angelicae Sinensis (*Dang Gui*)
    e. Rhizoma Curculiginis Orchioidis (*Xian Mao*)

    Answer: ___

502. Which is not an ingredient in _Bu Zhong Yi Qi Tang_ (Supplement the Center & Boost the Qi Decoction):
  a. Radix Codonopsitis Pilosulae (_Dang Shen_)
  b. Radix Astragali Membranacei (_Huang Qi_)
  c. Pericarpium Citri Reticulatae (_Chen Pi_)
  d. Radix Albus Paeoniae Lactiflorae (_Bai Shao_)
  e. Radix Angelicae Sinensis (_Dang Gui_)

  Answer: ___

503. Which formula is best for treating a defensive qi vacuity:
  a. _Dang Gui Liu Huang Tang_ (Dang Gui Six Yellows Decoction)
  b. _Gan Mai Da Zao Tang_ (Licorice, Wheat & Red Dates Decoction)
  c. _Yu Ping Feng San_ (Jade Windscreen Powder)
  d. _Ba Zhen Tang_ (Eight Pearls Decoction)
  e. _Shi Quan Da Bu Tang_ (Ten [Ingredients] Completely & Greatly Supplementing Decoction)

  Answer: ___

504. _Ma Xing Shi Gan Tang_ (Ephedra, Armeniaca, Gypsum & Licorice Decoction) treats coughing and panting due to:
  a. Phlegm rheum
  b. Phlegm cold
  c. Lung heat
  d. External contraction of wind heat
  e. None of the above

  Answer: ___

505. What is Radix Glycyrrhizae (_Gan Cao_)'s function within _Ma Xing Shi Gan Tang_ (Ephedra, Armeniaca, Gypsum & Licorice Decoction):
  a. Clears heat and resolves toxins
  b. Supplements the spleen and nourishes the heart
  c. Harmonizes all the other medicinals
  d. All of the above
  e. None of the above

  Answer: ___

506. What are Herba Ephedrae (_Ma Huang_) and Semen Pruni Armeniacae (_Xing Ren_)'s functions within _Ma Xing Shi Gan Tang_ (Ephedra, Armeniaca, Gypsum & Licorice Decoction):
  a. Clear heat and drain the lungs
  b. Diffuse the lungs and downbear counterflow
  c. Transform phlegm and scatter nodulation
  d. All of the above
  e. None of the above

  Answer: ___

507. What are Cortex Magnoliae Officinalis (*Hou Po*) and Fructus Immaturus Citri Aurantii (*Zhi Shi*)'s functions within *Da Cheng Qi Tang* (Major Order the Qi Decoction):
    a. Clear heat and disperse accumulation
    b. Abduct food and disperse stagnation
    c. Move the qi and relieve fullness
    d. Precipitate downward and free the flow of the stools
    e. None of the above

    Answer: ___

508. What are Radix Panacis Ginseng (*Ren Shen*), Fructus Zizyphi Jujubae (*Da Zao*), and Radix Glycyrrhizae (*Gan Cao*)'s functions within *Xiao Chai Hu Tang* (Minor Bupleurum Decoction):
    a. Transform phlegm and stop coughing
    b. Fortify the spleen and support the righteous
    c. Clear heat and resolve toxins
    d. Dispel wind and scatter cold
    e. None of the above

    Answer: ___

509. What is the function of Radix Albus Paeoniae Lactiflorae (*Bai Shao*) in *Si Ni San* (Four Counterflows Powder):
    a. Nourishes the blood to harmonize the liver
    b. Levels the liver and subdues yang
    c. Astringes yin and stops sweating
    d. Clears heat and quickens the blood
    e. None of the above

    Answer: ___

510. What are Radix Bupleuri (*Chai Hu*) and Herba Menthae Haplocalycis (*Bo He*)'s functions in *Xiao Yao San* (Rambling Powder):
    a. Course the liver and rectify the qi
    b. Clear heat and resolve depression
    c. Dispel wind and clear heat
    d. Open the nasal orifices
    e. None of the above

    Answer: ___

511. What are Gypsum Fibrosum (*Shi Gao*) and Rhizoma Anemarrhenae Aspheloidis (*Zhi Mu*)'s functions in *Bai Hu Tang* (White Tiger Decoction):
    a. Clear heat and resolve toxins
    b. Clear heat and precipitate downward
    c. Clear heat and transform phlegm
    d. Clear heat and enrich yin
    e. None of the above

    Answer: ___

512. The textbook pulse associated with *Huang Lian Jie Du Tang* (Coptis Resolve Toxins Decoction) is:
    a. Rapid and fine
    b. Fine and moderate or relaxed
    c. Rapid and forceful
    d. Bowstring and fine
    e. Soggy

    Answer: ___

513. The combination of Rhizoma Coptidis Chinensis (*Huang Lian*), Radix Scutellariae Baicalensis (*Huang Qin*), and Cortex Phellodendri (*Huang Bai*) in the above formula clears heat from:
    a. The upper burner .
    b. The upper and middle burners
    c. All three burners
    d. The middle and lower burners
    e. The upper and lower burners

    Answer: ___

514. *Pu Ji Xiao Du Yin* (Universal Benefit Disperse Toxins Drink) mainly treats:
    a. Cough
    b. Herpes zoster lesions in the rib-side
    c. Herpes genitalia lesions
    d. Athletes foot (a.k.a. Hong Kong foot)
    e. Sore, swollen, dry throat

    Answer: ___

515. The textbook pulse associated with *Long Dan Xie Gan Tang* (Gentiana Drain the Liver Decoction) is:
    a. Bowstring, fine, and rapid
    b. Bowstring, slippery, and rapid
    c. Slippery, surging, and rapid
    d. Floating, fine, and rapid
    e. Floating, large, and rapid

    Answer: ___

516. *Long Dan Xie Gan Tang* (Gentiana Drain the Liver Decoction) treats:
    a. Damp heat pouring downward
    b. Spleen vacuity engendering dampness and heat
    c. Damp heat with concomitant yin vacuity
    d. Damp heat with concomitant yang vacuity
    e. All of the above

    Answer: ___

517. What are the functions of Radix Angelicae Sinensis (*Dang Gui*) and uncooked Radix Rehmanniae (*Sheng Di*) within *Long Dan Xie Gan Tang* (Gentiana Drain the Liver Decoction):
    a. Cool the blood and stop bleeding
    b. Quicken the blood and dispel stasis
    c. Prevent windy medicinals from damaging yin
    d. All of the above
    e. A & C only

    Answer: ____

518. *Xie Bai San* (Drain the White Powder) treats:
    a. Cough due to consumption of yin by heat in the lungs
    b. Cough due to phlegm heat
    c. Cough due to phlegm cold
    d. Cough due to phlegm rheum
    e. Cough due to liver depression/depressive heat

    Answer: ____

519. *Bai Tou Weng Tang* (Pulsatilla Decoction) mainly treats:
    a. Heat accumulation constipation
    b. Damp heat strangury
    c. Damp heat diarrhea and dysentery
    d. Damp heat skin lesions
    e. All of the above

    Answer: ____

520. *Qing Shu Yi Qi Tang* (Clear Summerheat & Boost the Qi Decoction) treats:
    a. Qi and blood vacuity due to spleen vacuity
    b. Dampness and phlegm due to spleen vacuity
    c. Damp heat pouring downward
    d. Wind heat external contraction
    e. Qi and yin vacuity due to damage by summerheat

    Answer: ____

521. *Gui Pi Tang* (Restore the Spleen Decoction) treats:
    a. Bleeding due to spleen qi vacuity and depressive heat
    b. Bleeding due to spleen qi vacuity and blood stasis
    c. Bleeding due to spleen qi-kidney yang vacuity
    d. Bleeding due to spleen qi vacuity
    e. All of the above

    Answer: ____

522. *Yi Guan Jian* (One Link Decoction) treats:
    a. Liver blood-kidney yang vacuity
    b. Liver blood-kidney yin vacuity
    c. Liver-kidney yin vacuity with liver depression
    d. Liver depression-depressive heat
    e. Liver depression-kidney yang vacuity

    Answer: ___

523. Fructus Schisandrae Chinensis (*Wu Wei Zi*) and Semen Myristicae Fragrantis (*Rou Dou Kou*)'s functions within *Si Shen Wan* (Four Spirits Pills) are to:
    a. Fortify the spleen and supplement the kidneys
    b. Warm the middle and invigorate yang
    c. Secure the intestines and stop diarrhea
    d. Move the qi and stop pain
    e. None of the above

    Answer: ___

524. Which medicinal within *Suan Zao Ren Tang* (Zizyphus Spinosa Decoction) enable it to treat fever due to teething:
    a. Semen Zizyphi Spinosae (*Suan Zao Ren*)
    b. Radix Glycyrrhizae (*Gan Cao*)
    c. Radix Ligustici Wallichii (*Chuan Xiong*)
    d. Sclerotium Poriae Cocos (*Fu Ling*)
    e. Rhizoma Anemarrhenae Aspheloidis (*Zhi Mu*)

    Answer: ___

525. Zhu Dan-xi posited six depressions. Which one doesn't *Yue Ju Wan* (Escape Restraint Pills) treat:
    a. Qi
    b. Blood
    c. Heat
    d. Dampness
    e. Food
    f. Phlegm

    Answer: ___

526. What is the function of Herba Sargassii (*Hai Zao*), Thallus Algae (*Kun Bu*), Semen Citri Reticulatae (*Ju He*) within *Ju He Wan* (Orange Seed Pills):
    a. Scatter nodulation
    b. Soften the hard
    c. Move the qi
    d. Transform phlegm
    e. None of the above

    Answer: ___

527. *Ding Chuan Tang* (Stabilize Panting Decoction) is mainly for the treatment of:
   a. Panting and coughing during the acute or active stage
   b. Panting and coughing during the remission stage

   Answer: ___

528. Which is the best formula for treating nausea and vomiting during pregnancy due to liver depression/depressive heat and loss of stomach harmony:
   a. *Si Jun Zi Tang* (Four Gentlemen Decoction)
   b. *Liu Jun Zi Tang* (Six Gentlemen Decoction)
   c. *Ban Xia Hou Po Tang* (Pinellia & Magnolia Decoction)
   d. *Ju Pi Zhu Ru Tang* (Orange Peel & Bamboo Shaving Decoction)
   e. *Mai Men Dong Tang* (Ophiopogon Decoction)

   Answer: ___

529. *Bu Yang Huan Wu Tang* (Supplement Yang & Recover the Five [Viscera] Decoction) mainly treats:
   a. Blood stasis due to traumatic injury
   b. Blood stasis in the rib-side
   c. Blood stasis complicated by damp heat
   d. Blood stasis as the sequellae of wind stroke
   e. All of the above

   Answer: ___

530. *Wen Jing Tang* (Warm the Channels [or Menses] Decoction) treats:
   a. Only cold
   b. Only heat
   c. Only repletion
   d. Only vacuity
   e. Mixed hot and cold, vacuity and repletion

   Answer: ___

531. Tuber Ophiopogonis Japonici (*Mai Men Dong*)'s function within *Wen Jing Tang* (Warm the Channels [or Menses] Decoction) is to:
   a. Engender fluids and quicken the blood
   b. Engender fluids and loosen the chest
   c. Engender fluids and clear the heart
   d. Engender fluids and cool the blood
   e. Engender fluids and scatter nodulations

   Answer: ___

532. Fructus Germinatus Hordei Vulgaris (*Mai Ya*)'s function within *Zhen Gan Xi Feng Tang* (Settle the Liver & Extinguish Wind Decoction) is to:
    a. Prevent the heavy mineral medicinals from damaging the stomach
    b. Course the liver and rectify the qi
    c. Both of the above
    d. None of the above

    Answer: ___

533. Ramulus Cinnamomi Cassiae (*Gui Zhi*)'s function within *Wu Ling San* (Five [Ingredients] Poria Powder) is to:
    a. Quicken the blood and transform stasis
    b. Promote the bladder's qi transformation
    c. Dispel wind and scatter cold
    d. Fortify the spleen and transform dampness
    e. None of the above

    Answer: ___

534. If there is concomitant jaundice and edema, which two medicinals might you add to *Wu Ling San* (Five [Ingredients] Poria Powder):
    a. Herba Agastachis Seu Pogostemi (*Huo Xiang*) & Folium Perillae Frutescentis (*Zi Su Ye*)
    b. Radix Scutellariae Baicalensis (*Huang Qin*) & Rhizoma Coptidis Chinensis (*Huang Lian*)
    c. Radix Rubrus Paeoniae Lactiflorae (*Chi Shao*) & Radix Angelicae Sinensis (*Dang Gui*)
    d. Herba Artemisiae Capillaris (*Yin Chen Hao*) & Fructus Gardeniae Jasminoidis (*Shan Zhi Zi*)
    e. Fructus Cardamomi (*Bai Dou Kou*) & Fructus Amomi (*Sha Ren*)

    Answer: ___

535. Which is the best formula for wind phlegm one-sided (*i.e.*, migrainous) headache:
    a. *Tian Ma Gou Teng Yin* (Gastrodia & Uncaria Drink)
    b. *Ban Xia Bai Zhu Tian Ma Tang* (Pinellia, Atractylodes & Gastrodia Decoction)
    c. *Dan Zhi Xiao Yao San* (Moutan & Gardeniae Rambling Powder)
    d. *Chuan Xiong Cha Tiao San* (Ligusticum & Tea Mixed Powder)
    e. *Tao Ren Si Wu Tang* (Persica & Carthamus Four Materials Decoction)

    Answer: ___

536. *Wu Mei Wan* (Mume Pills) treats:
    a. Only cold patterns
    b. Only heat patterns
    c. Only repletion patterns
    d. Only vacuity patterns
    e. Mixed heat and cold, vacuity and repletion

    Answer: ___

537. Within *Wu Mei Wan* (Mume Pills), Radix Angelicae Sinensis (*Dang Gui*):
    a. Nourishes the blood
    b. Quickens the blood
    c. Cools the blood
    d. A & B
    e. B & C

    Answer: ___

Additions & Subtractions (*Jia Jian*)

538. What two medicinals are added to *Si Jun Zi Tang* (Four Gentlemen Decoction) when spleen qi vacuity gives rise to phlegm dampness:
    a. Pericarpium Citri Reticulatae (*Chen Pi*) & Rhizoma Pinelliae Ternatae (*Ban Xia*)
    b. Pericarpium Citri Reticulatae (*Chen Pi*) & Fructus Amomi (*Sha Ren*)
    c. Fructus Amomi (*Sha Ren*) & Radix Auklandiae Lappae (*Mu Xiang*)
    d. Radix Auklandiae Lappae (*Mu Xiang*) & Semen Arecae Catechu (*Bing Lang*)
    e. Radix Auklandiae Lappae (*Mu Xiang*) & Rhizoma Coptidis Chinensis (*Huang Lian*)

    Answer: ___

539. Which medicinal may be substituted for Rhizoma Pinelliae Ternatae (*Ban Xia*) in *Xiao Chai Hu Tang* (Minor Bupleurum Decoction) if there is thirst:
    a. Radix Trichosanthis Kirlowii (*Tian Hua Fen*)
    b. Radix Platycodi Grandiflori (*Jie Geng*)
    c. Radix Peucedani (*Qian Hu*)
    d. Radix Pseudostellariae (*Tai Zi Shen*)
    e. Bulbus Fritillariae Thunbergii (*Zhe Bei Mu*)

    Answer: ___

540. For yin vacuity thirsting and wasting with polyuria, which of the following medicinals should be removed from *Liu Wei Di Huang Wan* (Six Flavors Rehmannia Pills) and replaced with Radix Trichosanthis Kirlowii (*Tian Hua Fen*):
    a. cooked Radix Rehmanniae (*Shu Di*)
    b. Cortex Radicis Moutan (*Dan Pi*)
    c. Rhizoma Alismatis (*Ze Xie*)
    d. Radix Dioscoreae Oppositae (*Shan Yao*)
    e. Fructus Corni Officinalis (*Shan Zhu Yu*)

    Answer: ___

541. For liver blood-kidney yin vacuity low back pain, add which two ingredients to *Liu Wei Di Huang Wan* (Six Flavors Rehmannia Pills):
    a. Radix Morindae Officinalis (*Ba Ji Tian*) & Radix Dipsaci (*Xu Duan*)
    b. Radix Dipsaci (*Xu Duan*) & Herba Epimedii (*Xian Lian Pi*)
    c. Cortex Eucommiae Ulmoidis (*Du Zhong*) & Radix Achyranthis Bidentatae (*Niu Xi*)
    d. Herba Epimedii (*Xian Ling Pi*) & Rhizoma Curculiginis Orchioidis (*Xian Mao*)
    e. Radix Morindae Officinalis (*Ba Ji Tian*) & Cortex Cinnamomi Cassiae (*Rou Gui*)

    Answer: ___

542. For kidney yin vacuity with concomitant qi vacuity, add which two ingredients to *Liu Wei Di Huang Wan* (Six Flavors Rehmannia Pills):
    a. Radix Astragali Membranacei (*Huang Qi*) & Radix Angelicae Sinensis (*Dang Gui*)
    b. Radix Angelicae Sinensis (*Dang Gui*) & Radix Albus Paeoniae Lactiflorae (*Bai Shao*)
    c. Radix Platycodi Grandiflori (*Jie Geng*) & Bulbus Fritillariae Thunbergii (*Zhe Bei Mu*)
    d. Radix Panacis Ginseng (*Ren Shen*) & Radix Astragali Membranacei (*Huang Qi*)
    e. Radix Epimedii (*Xian Ling Pi*) & Rhizoma Curculiginis Orchioidis (*Xian Mao*)

    Answer: ___

543. For kidney yin vacuity with concomitant damp heat and painful, dribbling urination, increase the dosages of which two ingredients in *Liu Wei Di Huang Wan* (Six Flavors Rehmannia Pills):
    a. Sclerotium Poriae Cocos (*Fu Ling*) & Radix Dioscoreae Oppositae (*Shan Yao*)
    b. Sclerotium Poriae Cocos (*Fu Ling*) & Rhizoma Alismatis (*Ze Xie*)
    c. Radix Dioscoreae Oppositae (*Shan Yao*) & Fructus Corni Officinalis (*Shan Zhu Yu*)
    d. cooked Radix Rehmanniae (*Shu Di*) & Cortex Radicis Moutan (*Dan Pi*)
    e. Fructus Corni Officinalis (*Shan Zhu Yu*) & Rhizoma Alismatis (*Ze Xie*)

    Answer: ___

544. Add which of the following pairs of medicinals to *Liu Wei Di Huang Wan* (Six Flavors Rehmannia Pills) if kidney yin vacuity is complicated by heat toxins:
    a. Radix Rubrus Paeoniae Lactiflorae (*Chi Shao*) & uncooked Radix Rehmanniae (*Sheng Di*)
    b. Radix Scutellariae Baicalensis (*Huang Qin*) & Rhizoma Coptidis Chinensis (*Huang Lian*)
    c. Radix Gentianae Scabrae (*Long Dan Cao*) & uncooked Radix Rehmanniae (*Sheng Di*)
    d. Cortex Radicis Lycii Chinensis (*Gou Qi Zi*) & Carapax Amydae Sinensis (*Bei Jia*)
    e. Fructus Forsythiae Suspensae (*Lian Qiao*) & Flos Lonicerae Japonicae (*Jin Yin Hua*)

    Answer: ___

545. Which pair of ingredients can be added to *Liu Wei Di Huang Wan* (Six Flavors Rehmannia Pills) to treat seminal emission:
    a. Concha Ostreae (*Mu Li*) & Herba Sargassii (*Hai Zao*)
    b. Herba Sargassii (*Hai Zao*) & Thallus Algae (*Kun Bu*)
    c. Spica Prunellae Vulgaris (*Xia Ku Cao*) & Radix Scrophulariae Ningpoensis (*Xuan Shen*)
    d. Concha Ostreae (*Mu Li*) & Fructus Schisandrae Chinensis (*Wu Wei Zi*)
    e. Fructus Schisandrae Chinensis (*Wu Wei Zi*) & Radix Polygalae Tenuifoliae (*Yuan Zhi*)

    Answer: ___

546. Which pair of ingredients can be added to *Tong Xie Yao Fang* (Painful Diarrhea Essential Formula) for painful diarrhea due to liver assailing the spleen complicated by hemafecia:
    a. Sclerotium Poriae Cocos (*Fu Ling*) & Semen Coicis Lachryma-jobi (*Yi Yi Ren*)
    b. Radix Bupleuri (*Chai Hu*) & Fructus Citri Aurantii (*Zhi Ke*)
    c. Fructus Terminaliae Chebulae (*He Zi*) & Semen Myristicae Fragrantis (*Rou Dou Kou*)
    d. Rhizoma Cimicifugae (*Sheng Ma*) & Radix Bupleuri (*Chai Hu*)
    e. Flos Immaturus Sophorae Japonicae (*Huai Hua Mi*) & Radix Sanguisorbae (*Di Yu*)

    Answer: ___

547. Which pair of ingredients can be added to *Tong Xie Yao Fang* (Painful Diarrhea Essential Formula) for painful diarrhea due to liver assailing the spleen complicated by extremely watery stools:
   a. Sclerotium Poriae Cocos (*Fu Ling*) & Semen Coicis Lachryma-jobi (*Yi Yi Ren*)
   b. Radix Bupleuri (*Chai Hu*) & Fructus Citri Aurantii (*Zhi Ke*)
   c. Fructus Terminaliae Chebulae (*He Zi*) & Semen Myristicae Fragrantis (*Rou Dou Kou*)
   d. Rhizoma Cimicifugae (*Sheng Ma*) & Radix Bupleuri (*Chai Hu*)
   e. Flos Immaturus Sophorae Japonicae (*Huai Hua Mi*) & Radix Sanguisorbae (*Di Yu*)

   Answer: ___

548. Which pair of ingredients can be added to *Tong Xie Yao Fang* (Painful Diarrhea Essential Formula) for painful diarrhea due to liver assailing the spleen complicated by chest and rib-side distention and pain:
   a. Sclerotium Poriae Cocos (*Fu Ling*) & Semen Coicis Lachryma-jobi (*Yi Yi Ren*)
   b. Radix Bupleuri (*Chai Hu*) & Fructus Citri Aurantii (*Zhi Ke*)
   c. Fructus Terminaliae Chebulae (*He Zi*) & Semen Myristicae Fragrantis (*Rou Dou Kou*)
   d. Rhizoma Cimicifugae (*Sheng Ma*) & Radix Bupleuri (*Chai Hu*)
   e. Flos Immaturus Sophorae Japonicae (*Huai Hua Mi*) & Radix Sanguisorbae (*Di Yu*)

   Answer: ___

549. Which pair of ingredients can be added to *Tong Xie Yao Fang* (Painful Diarrhea Essential Formula) for painful diarrhea due to liver assailing the spleen complicated by tenesmus due to central qi fall:
   a. Sclerotium Poriae Cocos (*Fu Ling*) & Semen Coicis Lachryma-jobi (*Yi Yi Ren*)
   b. Radix Bupleuri (*Chai Hu*) & Fructus Citri Aurantii (*Zhi Ke*)
   c. Fructus Terminaliae Chebulae (*He Zi*) & Semen Myristicae Fragrantis (*Rou Dou Kou*)
   d. Rhizoma Cimicifugae (*Sheng Ma*) & Radix Bupleuri (*Chai Hu*)
   e. Flos Immaturus Sophorae Japonicae (*Huai Hua Mi*) & Radix Sanguisorbae (*Di Yu*)

   Answer: ___

550. Which pair of ingredients can be added to *Tong Xie Yao Fang* (Painful Diarrhea Essential Formula) for painful diarrhea due to liver assailing the spleen complicated by dampness and heat:
   a. Sclerotium Poriae Cocos (*Fu Ling*) & Semen Coicis Lachryma-jobi (*Yi Yi Ren*)
   b. Radix Bupleuri (*Chai Hu*) & Fructus Citri Aurantii (*Zhi Ke*)
   c. Radix Pulsatillae Chinensis (*Bai Tou Weng*) & Rhizoma Coptidis Chinensis (*Huang Lian*)
   d. Rhizoma Cimicifugae (*Sheng Ma*) & Radix Bupleuri (*Chai Hu*)
   e. Flos Immaturus Sophorae Japonicae (*Huai Hua Mi*) & Radix Sanguisorbae (*Di Yu*)

   Answer: ___

551. Which pair of ingredients can be added to *Tong Xie Yao Fang* (Painful Diarrhea Essential Formula) for painful diarrhea due to liver assailing the spleen complicated by severe qi vacuity:
   a. Sclerotium Poriae Cocos (*Fu Ling*) & Semen Coicis Lachryma-jobi (*Yi Yi Ren*)
   b. Radix Bupleuri (*Chai Hu*) & Fructus Citri Aurantii (*Zhi Ke*)
   c. Radix Pulsatillae Chinensis (*Bai Tou Weng*) & Rhizoma Coptidis Chinensis (*Huang Lian*)
   d. Rhizoma Cimicifugae (*Sheng Ma*) & Radix Bupleuri (*Chai Hu*)
   e. Radix Codonopsitis Pilosulae (*Dang Shen*) & Radix Astragali Membranacei (*Huang Qi*)

   Answer: ___

552. Which pair of ingredients can be added to *Dang Gui Bu Xue Tang* (Dang Gui Supplement the Blood Decoction) when spontaneous ejection of blood (*i.e.*, epistaxis) is due to a combination of qi vacuity and blood heat:
  a. Herba Agrimoniae Pilosae (*Xian He Cao*) & Radix Rubiae Cordifoliae (*Qian Cao Gen*)
  b. Flos Immaturus Sophorae Japonicae (*Huai Hua Mi*) & Rhizoma Cimicifugae (*Sheng Ma*)
  c. Fructus Gardeniae Jasminoidis (*Shan Zhi Zi*) & Fructus Corni Officinalis (*Shan Zhu Yu*)
  d. Fructus Schisandrae Chinensis (*Wu Wei Zi*) & Fructus Pruni Mume (*Wu Mei*)
  e. Os Sepiae Seu Sepiellae (*Wu Zei Gu*) & Ootheca Mantidis (*Sang Piao Xiao*)

  Answer: ___

553. Which pair of medicinals can be added to *Si Wu Tang* (Four Materials Decoction) for the treatment of replete pattern stasis heat blocked menstruation (*i.e.*, amenorrhea):
  a. Radix Et Rhizoma Rhei (*Da Huang*) & Mirabilitum (*Mang Xiao*)
  b. Rhizoma Cyperi Rotundi (*Xiang Fu*) & Radix Linderae Strychnifoliae (*Wu Yao*)
  c. Cortex Cinnamomi Cassiae (*Rou Gui*) & Radix Lateralis Praeparatus Aconiti Carmichaeli (*Fu Zi*)
  d. Cortex Radicis Lycii Chinensis (*Di Gu Pi*) & Cortex Radicis Moutan (*Dan Pi*)
  e. Semen Pruni Persicae (*Tao Ren*) & Flos Carthami Tinctorii (*Hong Hua*)

  Answer: ___

554. Which pair of medicinals can be added to *Si Wu Tang* (Four Materials Decoction) for the treatment of cold congelation blocked menstruation (*i.e.*, amenorrhea):
  a. Radix Et Rhizoma Rhei (*Da Huang*) & Mirabilitum (*Mang Xiao*)
  b. Rhizoma Cyperi Rotundi (*Xiang Fu*) & Radix Linderae Strychnifoliae (*Wu Yao*)
  c. Cortex Cinnamomi Cassiae (*Rou Gui*) & Radix Lateralis Praeparatus Aconiti Carmichaeli (*Fu Zi*)
  d. Cortex Radicis Lycii Chinensis (*Di Gu Pi*) & Cortex Radicis Moutan (*Dan Pi*)
  e. Semen Pruni Persicae (*Tao Ren*), Flos Carthami Tinctorii (*Hong Hua*)

  Answer: ___

555. Which pair of medicinals can be added to *Si Wu Tang* (Four Materials Decoction) for the treatment of blood heat:
  a. Radix Scutellariae Baicalensis (*Huang Qin*) & Rhizoma Coptidis Chinensis (*Huang Lian*)
  b. Rhizoma Cyperi Rotundi (*Xiang Fu*) & Radix Linderae Strychnifoliae (*Wu Yao*)
  c. Cortex Cinnamomi Cassiae (*Rou Gui*) & Radix Lateralis Praeparatus Aconiti Carmichaeli (*Fu Zi*)
  d. Radix Codonopsitis Pilosulae (*Dang Shen*) & Radix Astragali Membranacei (*Huang Qi*)
  e. Semen Pruni Persicae (*Tao Ren*) & Flos Carthami Tinctorii (*Hong Hua*)

  Answer: ___

556. Which pair of medicinals can be added to *Bu Zhong Yi Qi Tang* (Supplement the Center & Boost the Qi Decoction) when spleen qi vacuity is complicated by vacuity heat:
  a. Radix Scutellariae Baicalensis (*Huang Qin*) & Rhizoma Coptidis Chinensis (*Huang Lian*)
  b. Cortex Phellodendri (*Huang Bai*) & Rhizoma Anemarrhenae Aspheloidis (*Zhi Mu*)
  c. Fructus Gardeniae Jasminoidis (*Shan Zhi Zi*) & Cortex Radicis Moutan (*Dan Pi*)
  d. Cortex Radicis Dictamni Dasycarpi (*Bai Xian Pi*) & Fructus Kochiae Scopariae (*Di Fu Zi*)
  e. None of the above

  Answer: ___

557. Which pair of medicinals can be added to *Bu Zhong Yi Qi Tang* (Supplement the Center & Boost the Qi Decoction) when spleen qi vacuity is complicated by kidney yang vacuity:
    a. Sclerotium Poriae Cocos (*Fu Ling*) & Semen Coicis Lachryma-jobi (*Yi Yi Ren*)
    b. Radix Dioscoreae Oppositae (*Shan Yao*) & Semen Dolichoris Lablab (*Bai Bian Dou*)
    c. Rhizoma Curculiginis Orchioidis (*Xian Mao*) & Herba Epimedii (*Xian Ling Pi*)
    d. Herba Ecliptae Prostratae (*Han Lian Cao*) & Fructus Ligustri Lucidi (*Nu Zhen Zi*)
    e. Fructus Corni Officinalis (*Shan Zhu Yu*) & Fructus Schisandrae Chinensis (*Wu Wei Zi*)

    Answer: ___

558. Which pair of medicinals can be added to *Bu Zhong Yi Qi Tang* (Supplement the Center & Boost the Qi Decoction) when spleen qi vacuity is complicated by kidney yin vacuity:
    a. Sclerotium Poriae Cocos (*Fu Ling*) & Semen Coicis Lachryma-jobi (*Yi Yi Ren*)
    b. Radix Dioscoreae Oppositae (*Shan Yao*) & Semen Dolichoris Lablab (*Bai Bian Dou*)
    c. Rhizoma Curculiginis Orchioidis (*Xian Mao*) & Herba Epimedii (*Xian Ling Pi*)
    d. Herba Ecliptae Prostratae (*Han Lian Cao*) & Fructus Ligustri Lucidi (*Nu Zhen Zi*)
    e. Fructus Corni Officinalis (*Shan Zhu Yu*) & Fructus Myristicae Fragrantis (*Rou Dou Kou*)

    Answer: ___

559. Which pair of medicinals can be added to *Bu Zhong Yi Qi Tang* (Supplement the Center & Boost the Qi Decoction) when spleen qi vacuity is complicated by kidney qi loss of securing:
    a. Sclerotium Poriae Cocos (*Fu Ling*) & Semen Coicis Lachryma-jobi (*Yi Yi Ren*)
    b. Radix Dioscoreae Oppositae (*Shan Yao*) & Semen Dolichoris Lablab (*Bai Bian Dou*)
    c. Rhizoma Curculiginis Orchioidis (*Xian Mao*) & Herba Epimedii (*Xian Ling Pi*)
    d. Herba Ecliptae Prostratae (*Han Lian Cao*) & Fructus Ligustri Lucidi (*Nu Zhen Zi*)
    e. Fructus Corni Officinalis (*Shan Zhu Yu*) & Fructus Myristicae Fragrantis (*Rou Dou Kou*)

    Answer: ___

560. Which pair of medicinals can be added to *Bu Zhong Yi Qi Tang* (Supplement the Center & Boost the Qi Decoction) when spleen qi vacuity is complicated by phlegm dampness:
    a. Sclerotium Poriae Cocos (*Fu Ling*) & Rhizoma Pinelliae Ternatae (*Ban Xia*)
    b. Radix Dioscoreae Oppositae (*Shan Yao*) & Semen Dolichoris Lablab (*Bai Bian Dou*)
    c. Rhizoma Curculiginis Orchioidis (*Xian Mao*) & Herba Epimedii (*Xian Ling Pi*)
    d. Herba Ecliptae Prostratae (*Han Lian Cao*) & Fructus Ligustri Lucidi (*Nu Zhen Zi*)
    e. Fructus Corni Officinalis (*Shan Zhu Yu*) & Fructus Myristicae Fragrantis (*Rou Dou Kou*)

    Answer: ___

561. Which pair of medicinals can be added to *Bu Zhong Yi Qi Tang* (Supplement the Center & Boost the Qi Decoction) when spleen qi vacuity is complicated by food stagnation:
    a. Sclerotium Poriae Cocos (*Fu Ling*) & Rhizoma Pinelliae Ternatae (*Ban Xia*)
    b. Massa Medica Fermentata (*Shen Qu*) & Fructus Crataegi (*Shan Zha*)
    c. Rhizoma Gastrodiae Elatae (*Tian Ma*) & Ramulus Uncariae Cum Uncis (*Gou Teng*)
    d. Herba Ecliptae Prostratae (*Han Lian Cao*) & Fructus Ligustri Lucidi (*Nu Zhen Zi*)
    e. Fructus Amomi (*Sha Ren*) & Fructus Cardamomi (*Bai Dou Kou*)

    Answer: ___

562. Which medicinals should be added to *Shao Yao Gan Cao Tang* (Peony & Licorice Decoction) for the treatment of peptic ulcers with stomach yin vacuity:
    a. dry Rhizoma Zingiberis (*Gan Jiang*) & Radix Astragali Membranacei (*Huang Qi*)
    b. Radix Glehniae Littoralis (*Sha Shen*) & Tuber Ophiopogonis (*Mai Men Dong*)
    c. Radix Salviae Miltiorrhizae (*Dan Shen*) & Radix Ligustici Wallichii (*Chuan Xiong*)
    d. Radix Bupleuri (*Chai Hu*) & Pericarpium Citri Reticulatae Viride (*Qing Pi*)
    e. None of the above

    Answer: ___

563. Which medicinals should be added to *Shao Yao Gan Cao Tang* (Peony & Licorice Decoction) for the treatment of peptic ulcers with liver depression qi stagnation:
    a. dry Rhizoma Zingiberis (*Gan Jiang*) & Radix Astragali Membranacei (*Huang Qi*)
    b. Radix Glehniae Littoralis (*Sha Shen*) & Tuber Ophiopogonis (*Mai Men Dong*)
    c. Radix Salviae Miltiorrhizae (*Dan Shen*) & Radix Ligustici Wallichii (*Chuan Xiong*)
    d. Radix Bupleuri (*Chai Hu*) & Pericarpium Citri Reticulatae Viride (*Qing Pi*)
    e. None of the above

    Answer: ___

564. Which medicinals should be added to *Shao Yao Gan Cao Tang* (Peony & Licorice Decoction) for the treatment of peptic ulcers with blood stasis:
    a. dry Rhizoma Zingiberis (*Gan Jiang*) & Radix Astragali Membranacei (*Huang Qi*)
    b. Radix Glehniae Littoralis (*Sha Shen*) & Tuber Ophiopogonis (*Mai Men Dong*)
    c. Radix Salviae Miltiorrhizae (*Dan Shen*) & Radix Ligustici Wallichii (*Chuan Xiong*)
    d. Radix Bupleuri (*Chai Hu*) & Pericarpium Citri Reticulatae Viride (*Qing Pi*)
    e. None of the above

    Answer: ___

565. Which medicinals should be added to *Shao Yao Gan Cao Tang* (Peony & Licorice Decoction) for the treatment of peptic ulcers with spleen-stomach vacuity cold:
    a. dry Rhizoma Zingiberis (*Gan Jiang*) & Radix Astragali Membranacei (*Huang Qi*)
    b. Radix Glehniae Littoralis (*Sha Shen*) & Tuber Ophiopogonis (*Mai Men Dong*)
    c. Radix Salviae Miltiorrhizae (*Dan Shen*) & Radix Ligustici Wallichii (*Chuan Xiong*)
    d. Radix Bupleuri (*Chai Hu*) & Pericarpium Citri Reticulatae Viride (*Qing Pi*)
    e. None of the above

    Answer: ___

566. Which medicinals should be added to *Xiao Yao San* (Rambling Powder) for the treatment of dizziness and vertigo:
    a. Rhizoma Gastrodiae Elatae (*Tian Ma*) & Ramulus Uncariae Cum Uncis (*Gou Teng*)
    b. Bulbus Fritillariae Thunbergii (*Zhe Bei Mu*) & Rhizoma Pinelliae Ternatae (*Ban Xia*)
    c. Radix Scutellariae Baicalensis (*Huang Qin*) & Rhizoma Pinelliae Ternatae (*Ban Xia*)
    d. Rhizoma Pinelliae Ternatae (*Ban Xia*) & Pericarpium Citri Reticulatae (*Chen Pi*)
    e. Caulis Bambusae In Taeniis (*Zhu Ru*) & Pericarpium Citri Reticulatae (*Chen Pi*)

    Answer: ___

567. Which medicinals should be added to *Xiao Yao San* (Rambling Powder) for the treatment of liver depression and spleen vacuity with phlegm dampness:
    a. Rhizoma Gastrodiae Elatae (*Tian Ma*) & Ramulus Uncariae Cum Uncis (*Gou Teng*)
    b. Pericarpium Citri Reticulatae (*Chen Pi*) & Ramulus Cinnamomi Cassiae (*Gui Zhi*)
    c. Radix Scutellariae Baicalensis (*Huang Qin*) & Rhizoma Pinelliae Ternatae (*Ban Xia*)
    d. Rhizoma Pinelliae Ternatae (*Ban Xia*) & Pericarpium Citri Reticulatae (*Chen Pi*)
    e. Caulis Bambusae In Taeniis (*Zhu Ru*) & Pericarpium Citri Reticulatae (*Chen Pi*)

    Answer: ___

568. Which medicinals should be added to *Xiao Yao San* (Rambling Powder) for the treatment of liver depression and spleen vacuity with nausea and vomiting:
    a. Rhizoma Gastrodiae Elatae (*Tian Ma*) & Ramulus Uncariae Cum Uncis (*Gou Teng*)
    b. Rhizoma Coptidis Chinensis (*Huang Lian*) & Ramulus Cinnamomi Cassiae (*Gui Zhi*)
    c. Radix Scutellariae Baicalensis (*Huang Qin*) & Rhizoma Pinelliae Ternatae (*Ban Xia*)
    d. Rhizoma Pinelliae Ternatae (*Ban Xia*) & Pericarpium Citri Reticulatae (*Chen Pi*)
    e. Caulis Bambusae In Taeniis (*Zhu Ru*) & Pericarpium Citri Reticulatae (*Chen Pi*)

    Answer: ___

569. Which medicinals should be added to *Xiao Yao San* (Rambling Powder) for the treatment of liver depression and spleen vacuity with depressive heat and phlegm in the stomach and lungs:
    a. Fructus Evodiae Rutecarpae (*Wu Zhu Yu*) & Rhizoma Coptidis Chinensis (*Huang Lian*)
    b. Rhizoma Coptidis Chinensis (*Huang Lian*) & Ramulus Cinnamomi Cassiae (*Gui Zhi*)
    c. Radix Scutellariae Baicalensis (*Huang Qin*) & Rhizoma Pinelliae Ternatae (*Ban Xia*)
    d. Rhizoma Pinelliae Ternatae (*Ban Xia*) & Pericarpium Citri Reticulatae (*Chen Pi*)
    e. Caulis Bambusae In Taeniis (*Zhu Ru*) & Pericarpium Citri Reticulatae (*Chen Pi*)

    Answer: ___

570. Which medicinals should be added to *Xiao Yao San* (Rambling Powder) for the treatment of liver depression and spleen-kidney dual vacuity with enduring dampness and heat abnormal vaginal discharge:
    a. Fructus Corni Officinalis (*Shan Zhu Yu*) & Fructus Schisandrae Chinensis (*Wu Wei Zi*)
    b. Fructus Gardeniae Jasminoidis (*Shan Zhi Zi*) & Cortex Radicis Moutan (*Dan Pi*)
    c. Radix Scutellariae Baicalensis (*Huang Qin*) & Rhizoma Pinelliae Ternatae (*Ban Xia*)
    d. Rhizoma Pinelliae Ternatae (*Ban Xia*) & Semen Coicis Lachryma-jobi (*Yi Yi Ren*)
    e. Radix Dioscoreae Oppositae (*Shan Yao*) & Semen Euryalis Ferocis (*Qian Shi*)

    Answer: ___

571. Which medicinals should be added to *Xiao Yao San* (Rambling Powder) for the treatment of liver depression and spleen vacuity with abdominal distention, lack of appetite, and bad breath:
    a. Fructus Germinatus Hordei Vulgaris (*Mai Ya*) & Fructus Amomi (*Sha Ren*)
    b. Fructus Evodiae Rutecarpae (*Wu Zhu Yu)* & Rhizoma Coptidis Chinensis (*Huang Lian*)
    c. Pericarpium Citri Reticulatae (*Chen Pi*) & Rhizoma Pinelliae Ternatae (*Ban Xia*)
    d. Rhizoma Pinelliae Ternatae (*Ban Xia*) & Semen Coicis Lachryma-jobi (*Yi Yi Ren*)
    e. Radix Dioscoreae Oppositae (*Shan Yao*) & Semen Euryalis Ferocis (*Qian Shi*)

    Answer: ___

Categorizing

572. Radix Bupleuri (*Chai Hu*) is usually categorized as what type of medicinal:
    a. Qi-rectifier
    b. Acrid, warm exterior-resolver
    c. Acrid, cool exterior-resolver
    d. Harmonizer
    e. Blood-rectifier

    Answer: ___

573. *Xiao Chai Hu Tang* (Minor Bupleurum Decoction) is usually categorized as what type of formula:
    a. Qi-rectifying
    b. Qi-supplementing
    c. Blood-rectifying
    d. Heat-clearing
    e. Harmonizing

    Answer: ___

574. *Si Wu Tang* (Four Materials Decoction) is usually categorized as what type of formula:
    a. Blood-supplementing
    b. Blood-quickening
    c. Blood-cooling
    d. Orifice-opening
    e. Downward precipitating

    Answer: ___

575. Fructus Pruni Mume (*Wu Mei*) is usually categorized as what type of medicinal:
    a. Worm-dispeller
    b. Astringent
    c. Yin-enricher
    d. Phlegm-transformer
    e. Heat-clearer

    Answer: ___

576. Semen Ginkgonis Bilobae (*Bai Guo*) is usually categorized as what type of medicinal:
    a. Worm-dispeller
    b. Astringent
    c. Yin-enricher
    d. Phlegm-transformer
    e. Heat-clearer

    Answer: ___

577. Uncooked Radix Rehmanniae (*Sheng Di*) is usually categorized as what type of medicinal:
    a. Worm-dispeller
    b. Astringent
    c. Yin-enricher
    d. Phlegm-transformer
    e. Heat-clearer

    Answer: ___

578. Dry Rhizoma Zingiberis (*Gan Jiang*) is usually categorized as what type of medicinal:
    a. Worm-dispeller
    b. Interior-warmer
    c. Yin-enricher
    d. Phlegm-transformer
    e. Heat-clearer

    Answer: ___

579. *Wu Mei Wan* (Mume Pills) is usually categorized as what kind of formula:
    a. Qi-supplementing
    b. Qi-rectifying
    c. Blood-supplementing
    d. Worm-dispelling
    e. Dampness-eliminating

    Answer: ___

580. *Ban Xia Xie Xin Tang* (Pinellia Drain the Heart Decoction) is usually categorized as what kind of formula:
    a. Qi-supplementing
    b. Qi-rectifying
    c. Harmonizing
    d. Heat-clearing
    e. Dampness-eliminating

    Answer: ___

581. *Tian Ma Gou Teng Yin* (Gastrodia & Uncaria Drink) is usually categorized as what kind of formula:
    a. Qi-supplementing
    b. Qi-rectifying
    c. Harmonizing
    d. Heat-clearing
    e. Wind-extinguishing

    Answer: ___

582. Cooked Radix Rehmanniae (*Shu Di*) is usually categorized as what kind of medicinal:
    a. Heat-clearing
    b. Blood-supplementing
    c. Blood-quickening
    d. Fluid-engendering
    e. None of the above

    Answer: ___

583. Rhizoma Cyperi Rotundi (*Xiang Fu*) is usually categorized as what kind of medicinal:
    a. Blood-quickening
    b. Qi-rectifier
    c. Exterior-resolver
    d. Wind damp treating
    e. Wind-extinguishing

    Answer: ___

584. Radix Dioscoreae Oppositae (*Shan Yao*) is usually categorized as what kind of medicinal:
    a. Qi-supplementing
    b. Yin-supplementing
    c. Yang-supplementing
    d. Damp-eliminating
    e. Wind damp treating

    Answer: ___

585. Sclerotium Poriae Cocos (*Fu Ling*) is usually categorized as what kind of medicinal:
    a. Spirit-quieting
    b. Qi-supplementing
    c. Damp-eliminating
    d. Phlegm-transforming
    e. Yang-supplementing

    Answer: ___

586. Herba Menthae Haplocalycis (*Bo He*) is usually categorized as what kind of medicinal:
    a. Acrid, warm exterior-resolver
    b. Acrid, cool exterior-resolver
    c. Qi-rectifier
    d. Heat-clearing
    e. Wind damp treating

    Answer: ___

587. Fructus Terminaliae Chebulae (*He Zi*) is usually categorized as what kind of medicinal:
    a. Worm-killing
    b. Damp-eliminating
    c. Qi-supplementing
    d. Securing and astringing
    e. None of the above

    Answer: ___

588. Fructus Meliae Toosendan (*Chuan Lian Zi*) is usually categorized as what kind of medicinal:
    a. Worm-killing
    b. Heat-clearing
    c. Qi-supplementing
    d. Blood-quickening
    e. Qi-rectifier

    Answer: ___

589. Fructus Ligustri Lucidi (*Nu Zhen Zi*) is usually categorized as what kind of medicinal:
    a. Yang-supplementing
    b. Yin-supplementing
    c. Stop bleeding
    d. Qi-supplementing
    e. Heat-clearing

    Answer: ___

590. Fructus Corni Officinalis (*Shan Zhu Yu*) is usually categorized as what kind of medicinal:
    a. Securing and astringing
    b. Yang-supplementing
    c. Yin-supplementing
    d. Qi-supplementing
    e. Damp-eliminating

    Answer: ___

591. Semen Cuscutae Chinensis (*Tu Si Zi*) is usually categorized as what kind of medicinal:
    a. Securing and astringing
    b. Yang-supplementing
    c. Yin-supplementing
    d. Qi-supplementing
    e. Damp-eliminating

    Answer: ___

592. Ramulus Uncariae Cum Uncis (*Gou Teng*) is usually categorized as what kind of medicinal:
    a. Heat-clearing
    b. Qi-rectifying
    c. Wind-extinguishing
    d. Blood-quickening
    e. Phlegm-transforming

    Answer: ___

593. Cortex Radicis Acanthopanacis Gracilistyli (*Wu Jia Pi*) is usually categorized as what kind of medicinal:
    a. Qi-supplementing
    b. Blood-supplementing
    c. Yin-supplementing
    d. Yang-supplementing
    e. Wind damp treating

    Answer: ___

594. Galla Rhois (*Wu Bei Zi*) is usually categorized as what kind of medicinal:
    a. Worm-killing
    b. External application
    c. Securing and astringing
    d. Heat-clearing
    e. Blood-quickening

    Answer: ___

Treatment Principles (*Zhi Li*)

595. If one's treatment principles are to course the liver and rectify the qi, then one should look for one's guiding formula under what category:
    a. Qi-rectifying
    b. Blood-rectifying
    c. Heat-clearing
    d. Dampness-eliminating
    e. Worm-dispelling

    Answer: ___

596. If one's treatment principles are to fortify the spleen and boost the qi, one should look for their guiding formula under which category:
    a. Yang-supplementing
    b. Qi-rectifying
    c. Phlegm-transforming
    d. Qi-supplementing
    e. Blood-supplementing

    Answer: ___

597. If one's treatment principles are to course the liver and rectify the qi, fortify the spleen and boost the qi, one should look for their guiding formula under which category:
    a. Yang-supplementing
    b. Qi-rectifying
    c. Phlegm-transforming
    d. Qi-supplementing
    e. Harmonizing

    Answer: ___

598. If one's treatment principles are to fortify the spleen and clear heat and dampness from the stomach and intestines, one should look for their guiding formula under which category:
    a. Yang-supplementing
    b. Qi-rectifying
    c. Phlegm-transforming
    d. Qi-supplementing
    e. Harmonizing

    Answer: ___

599. If one's treatment principles are to resolve the exterior and clear heat, one should look for their guiding formula under which category:
    a. Acrid, warm exterior-resolving
    b. Acrid, cool exterior-resolving
    c. Phlegm-transforming
    d. Qi-supplementing
    e. Harmonizing

    Answer: ___

600. If the pattern is one of spleen qi vacuity, the treatment principles are to:
    a. Fortify the spleen and supplement the qi
    b. Arouse the spleen and dry dampness
    c. Clear the spleen and drain the qi
    d. Upbear the spleen and downbear turbidity
    e. None of the above

    Answer: ___

601. If the pattern is one of liver depression qi stagnation, the treatment principles are to:
    a. Harmonize the liver and downbear the qi
    b. Course the liver and rectify the qi
    c. Course the liver and clear heat
    d. Clear heat and resolve depression
    e. Emolliate the liver and nourish yin

    Answer: ___

602. If the pattern is one of kidney yang vacuity, the treatment principles are to:
    a. Supplement the kidneys and enrich yin
    b. Supplement the kidneys and secure and astringe
    c. Supplement the kidneys and grasp or absorb the qi
    d. Supplement the kidneys and invigorate yang
    e. Dispel wind and scatter cold

    Answer: ___

603. If the pattern is one of phlegm nodulation, the treatment principles are to:
    a. Clear heat and transform phlegm
    b. Transform phlegm and scatter cold
    c. Transform phlegm and scatter nodulation
    d. Break the qi and soften the hard
    e. None of the above

    Answer: ___

604. If the pattern is one of blood vacuity with damp heat, the treatment principles are to:
    a. Supplement the blood, clear heat and resolve toxins
    b. Clear heat and eliminate dampness, supplement the blood
    c. Supplement the blood, clear heat and eliminate dampness
    d. Clear heat and cool the blood
    e. Clear heat and stop bleeding

    Answer: ___

605. If the pattern is one of spleen-kidney dual vacuity, the treatment principles are to:
    a. Fortify the spleen and supplement the qi, supplement the kidneys and invigorate yang
    b. Fortify the spleen and supplement the kidneys, secure and astringe
    c. Supplement the spleen and kidneys, warm yang and seep dampness
    d. Supplement the spleen and kidneys, warm yang and dispel stasis
    e. None of the above

    Answer: ___

606. If the pattern is one of damp heat stasis and stagnation, the treatment principles are to:
    a. Clear heat and resolve toxins, cool the blood and dispel stasis
    b. Clear heat and eliminate dampness, transform food and disperse stagnation
    c. Clear heat and eliminate dampness, disperse stagnation and dispel stasis
    d. Disperse stagnation and dispel stasis, clear heat and resolve toxins
    e. Supplement the spleen and boost the qi, clear heat and quicken the blood

    Answer: ___

Case History Questions

607. Your patient has bodily aches and pains, aversion to cold, a very high temperature but no perspiration, a floating (*fu*), tight (*jin*) pulse, and a cough. You prescribe:
   a. *Da Qing Long Tang* (Major Blue-green Dragon Decoction)
   b. *Gui Zhi Tang* (Cinnamon Twig Decoction)
   c. *Xiao Qing Long Tang* (Minor Blue-green Dragon Decoction)
   d. *Sheng Mai San* (Engender the Vessels [or Pulse] Powder)
   e. None of the above

   Answer: ___

608. Your patient has bodily aches and pain, aversion to cold, emission of heat but no sweating, a floating (*fu*), tight (*jin*) pulse, and especially tight, painful neck and shoulders. You prescribe:
   a. *Da Qing Long Tang* (Major Blue-green Dragon Decoction)
   b. *Gui Zhi Tang* (Cinnamon Twig Decoction)
   c. *Xiao Qing Long Tang* (Minor Blue-green Dragon Decoction)
   d. *Ge Gen Tang* (Pueraria Decoction)
   e. *Ma Huang Tang* (Ephedra Decoction)

   Answer: ___

609. Your patient has premenstrual breast distention and pain, irritability, a tendency to cry, and acne around her chin and mouth. Her tongue is red with slightly yellow fur, and her pulse is bowstring and slightly rapid. Her pattern discrimination in terms of the premenstrual acne is:
   a. Liver depression qi stagnation
   b. Qi stagnation and blood stasis
   c. Heat toxins
   d. Depressive heat in her lungs and stomach
   e. Phlegm nodulation

   Answer: ___

610. The best guiding formula for the above patient is:
   a. *Xiao Yao San* (Rambling Powder)
   b. *Dan Zhi Xiao Yao San* (Moutan & Gardeniae Rambling Powder)
   c. *Xiao Chai Hu Tang* (Minor Bupleurum Decoction)
   d. *Chai Hu Shu Gan Tang* (Bupleurum Course the Liver Decoction)
   e. *Chai Hu Gui Zhi Tang* (Bupleurum & Cinnamon Twig Decoction)

   Answer: ___

611. Which two medicinals should you add to the above formula if the acne lesions in the above case are quite painful and leave behind purple scars which take a long time to go away:
   a. Bulbus Fritillariae Thunbergii (*Zhe Bei Mu*) & Radix Scrophulariae Ningpoensis (*Xuan Shen*)
   b. Rhizoma Coptidis Chinensis (*Huang Lian*) & Herba Violae Yedoensis Cum Radice (*Zi Hua Di Ding*)
   c. Herba Ecliptae Prostratae (*Han Lian Cao*) & Fructus Ligustri Lucidi (*Nu Zhen Zi*)

d. Radix Rubrus Paeoniae Lactiflorae (*Chi Shao*) & Cortex Radicis Moutan (*Dan Pi*)

e. uncooked Radix Rehmanniae (*Sheng Di*) & Tuber Ophiopogonis Japonici (*Mai Men Dong*)

Answer: ___

612. Your patient has alternating fever and chills, a bad sore throat and cough with slightly yellow phlegm, fatigue, no appetite, yellow fur on one side of their tongue, and a bowstring pulse. Which formula do you prescribe:

a. *Gui Zhi Tang* (Cinnamon Twig Decoction)

b. *Bai Hu Tang* (White Tiger Decoction)

c. *Ma Xing Shi Gan Tang* (Ephedra, Armeniaca, Gypsum & Licorice Decoction)

d. *Xiao Yao San* (Rambling Powder)

e. *Xiao Chai Hu Tang* (Minor Bupleurum Decoction)

Answer: ___

613. Your patient has heavy uterine bleeding which is profuse in quantity but thin and watery in consistency. She is fatigued and dizzy when she stands up, and her bleeding is worse when she is fatigued. She is also extremely overweight. Her tongue is swollen and her pulse is fine and weak. Which formula do you prescribe:

a. *Er Chen Tang* (Two Aged [Ingredients] Decoction)

b. *Wen Dan Tang* (Warm the Gallbladder Decoction)

c. *Gui Pi Tang* (Restore the Spleen Decoction)

d. *Liu Jun Zi Tang* (Six Gentlemen Decoction)

e. *Bu Zhong Yi Qi Tang* (Supplement the Center & Boost the Qi Decoction)

Answer: ___

614. Your patient is three weeks old and has colic. Their abdomen is bloated and they pump their legs to their abdomen when they cry. Their face is red and their hands and feet are hot when they cry. Their breath is not sweet. When they are able to pass gas, their crying calms temporarily. Which formula do you prescribe:

a. *Bao He Wan* (Protect Harmony Decoction)

b. *Si Jun Zi Tang* (Four Gentlemen Decoction)

c. *Dao Chi San* (Abduct the Red Decoction)

d. *Suan Zao Ren Tang* (Zizyphus Spinosa Decoction)

e. *Da Cheng Qi Tang* (Major Order the Qi Decoction)

Answer: ___

615. Your patient has acne on their forehead. The lesion is light red and made up of many small red pimples which never really pustulate. This rash is spread evenly across the forehead. There is not pain, no deep nodulations, or purple scarring. Their tongue is light red with a red tip and scanty fur, and their pulse is fine and rapid. Their acne gets worse during and right after menstruation. Which formula do you prescribe:

a. *Xiao Chai Hu Tang* (Minor Bupleurum Decoction)

b. *Da Cheng Qi Tang* (Major Order the Qi Decoction)

c. *Zhi Bai Di Huang Wan* (Anemarrhena & Phellodendron Rehmannia Pills)
d. *Ma Xing Shi Gan Tang* (Ephedra, Armeniaca, Gypsum & Licorice Decoction)
e. *Er Chen Tang* (Two Aged [Ingredients] Decoction)

Answer: ___

616. Your patient has chronic colitis of many years duration. Right now they are having diarrhea with some bright red blood in their stools but no mucus. They are quite thirsty. They experience tidal heat and their tongue is dark red with scanty fur, and their pulse is surging and rapid. Besides enduring spleen qi vacuity, what other disease mechanisms are present:
a. Heat toxins
b. Depressive heat
c. Internal heat damaging yin fluids
d. Damp heat
e. None of the above

Answer: ___

617. Your patient's main complaint is severe menstrual pain. This occurs on day one of her menses. There is a combination of generalized cramps and sharp, stabbing, right-sided pain. In addition there is low back soreness and pain. The woman is 42 years old. She has a chronic, thick, white cheesy vaginal discharge often accompanied by burning urination and/or external vaginal itching and inflammation. Premenstrually, her breasts are swollen and sore, she is irritable and severely fatigued. Her stools tend to be loose and sometimes are a bright, light yellow in color. Sometimes her stools also feel acidic or burning around the anus. She feels she lacks strength, her feet are cold, and she has to get up at least once per night to urinate. For the last two years, she hasn't had much sexual desire. The quantity of the blood is medium. Its color is bright red, but it contains dark, purple-black clots. Her tongue is swollen and somewhat red with yellow, slimy fur at its root. Her pulse is rapid. It is also bowstring and slippery at the left bar. Bowstring, slippery, and deep in both cubits. And floating, fine, and slippery in the right bar. Both inch positions are floating, large, and slippery. What is her pattern discrimination:
a. Liver depression qi stagnation
b. Blood stasis
c. Damp heat
d. Spleen qi vacuity
e. Kidney yang vacuity
f. All of the above

Answer: ___

618. Your guiding formula for the above case is:
a. *Ge Xia Zhu Yu Tang* (Below the Diaphragm Dispel Stasis Decoction)
b. *Shao Fu Zhu Yu Tang* (Lower Abdomen Dispel Stasis Decoction)

c. *Tao Ren Si Wu Tang* (Persicae & Carthamus Four Materials Decoction)

d. *Dan Zhi Xiao Yao San* (Moutan & Gardenia Rambling Powder)

e. *Shi Xiao San* (Loose a Smile Powder)

Answer: ___

619. Which two ingredients could you add to the above formula for damp heat stasis and stagnation:

a. Rhizoma Pinelliae Ternatae (*Ban Xia*) & Radix Scutellariae Baicalensis (*Huang Qin*)

b. Herba Patriniae Heterophyllae Cum Radice (*Bai Jiang Cao*) & Caulis Sargentodoxae (*Hong Teng*)

c. Fructus Pruni Mume (*Wu Mei*) & Herba Taraxaci Mongolici Cum Radice (*Pu Gong Ying*)

d. Semen Coicis Lachryma-jobi (*Yi Yi Ren*) & Cortex Phellodendri (*Huang Bai*)

e. None of the above

Answer: ___

620. What two medicinals might you add to the above formula to supplement the spleen and boost the qi:

a. Rhizoma Atractylodis (*Cang Zhu*) & Semen Coicis Lachryma-jobi (*Yi Yi Ren*)

b. Rhizoma Pinelliae Ternatae (*Ban Xia*) & dry Rhizoma Zingiberis (*Gan Jiang*)

c. Radix Astragali Membranacei (*Huang Qi*) & Radix Codonopsitis Pilosulae (*Dang Shen*)

d. Radix Dipsaci (*Xu Duan*) & Ramulus Loranthi Seu Visci (*Sang Ji Sheng*)

e. None of the above

Answer: ___

621. What two medicinals might you add to the above formula to supplement the kidneys and strengthen the low back:

a. Cortex Cinnamomi Cassiae (*Rou Gui*) & Radix Lateralis Praeparatus Aconiti Carmichaeli (*Fu Zi*)

b. Flos Caryophylli (*Ding Xiang*) & Fructus Evodiae Rutecarpae (*Wu Zhu Yu*)

c. Cortex Eucommiae Ulmoidis (*Du Zhong*) & Radix Dipsaci (*Xu Duan*)

d. Ramulus Loranthi Seu Visci (*Sang Ji Sheng*) & Radix Achyranthis Bidentatae (*Niu Xi*)

e. None of the above

Answer: ___

622. Your patient's main complaint is insomnia. She is 35 years old and somewhat overweight. However, her body type is more *tai yang* than *tai yin*. When she goes to bed at night, she is disturbed by nightmares and often wakes from sleep in a fright. She has heart palpitations, profuse phlegm, a reddish tongue with slimy, yellow fur, a bitter taste in her mouth when she wakes in the morning, and a bowstring, slippery, rapid pulse. She seems timid and irritable at the same time and is easily startled. Her pattern discrimination is:

a. Phlegm heat gallbladder timidity

b. Depressive liver heat

c. Phlegm heat confounding the orifices of the heart

d. Heart fire disturbing the spirit

e. Phlegm dampness and liver depression

Answer: ___

623. The guiding formula in the above case is:
   a. *Er Chen Tang* (Two Aged [Ingredients] Decoction)
   b. *Huang Lian Wen Dan Tang* (Coptis Warm the Gallbladder Decoction)
   c. *Wen Dan Tang* (Warm the Gallbladder Decoction)
   d. *Huang Lian E Jiao Tang* (Coptis & Donkey Skin Glue Decoction)
   e. *Dan Zhi Xiao Yao San* (Moutan & Gardeniae Rambling Powder)

   Answer: ___

624. If the above case were complicated by spleen qi vacuity with marked fatigue, you might add:
   a. Radix Angelicae Sinensis (*Dang Gui*) & Radix Astragali Membranacei (*Huang Qi*)
   b. Semen Coicis Lachryma-jobi (*Yi Yi Ren*) & Rhizoma Atractylodis (*Cang Zhu*)
   c. Herba Ecliptae Prostratae (*Han Lian Cao*) & Fructus Ligustri Lucidi (*Nu Zhen Zi*)
   d. Semen Sinapis Albae (*Bai Jie Zi*) & Semen Raphani Sativi (*Lai Fu Zi*)
   e. Radix Astragali Membranacei (*Huang Qi*) & Radix Codonopsitis Pilosulae (*Dang Shen*)

   Answer: ___

625. Your patient has enduring bouts of diarrhea. His stools are loose and contain pieces of undigested food, but their color is dark brown and they are very smelly. He is medium in build. He complains of fatigue. His appetite is excessive and he seems to "burn food" quickly. His tongue is fat with teethmarks on its edges with slightly yellow, somewhat slimy fur. His pulse is slightly rapid. His right bar position is forceful, slippery and floating. His pattern discrimination is:
   a. Spleen qi vacuity
   b. Stomach heat
   c. Stomach and intestines dampness and heat
   d. Spleen damp heat
   e. A & B
   f. A & C

   Answer: ___

626. The guiding formula in the above case is:
   a. *Liu Jun Zi Tang* (Six Gentlemen Decoction)
   b. *Bu Zhong Yi Qi Tang* (Supplement the Center & Boost the Qi Decoction)
   c. *Xiao Chai Hu Tang* (Minor Bupleurum Decoction)
   d. *Ban Xia Xie Xin Tang* (Pinelliae Drain the Heart Decoction)
   e. *Huang Qin Huang Lian Ge Gen Tang* (Scutellaria, Coptis & Pueraria Decoction)

   Answer: ___

627. If there were signs and symptoms of concomitant heart vacuity, which ingredient in the above formula might be doubled or tripled:
   a. Rhizoma Coptidis Chinensis (*Huang Lian*)
   b. Radix Scutellariae Baicalensis (*Huang Qin*)
   c. Rhizoma Pinelliae Ternatae (*Ban Xia*)

d. dry Rhizoma Zingiberis (*Gan Jiang*)
e. mix-fried Radix Glycyrrhizae (*Gan Cao*)

Answer: ___

628. The patient is a 24 year-old female. Her major complaint is low blood pressure with cold hands and feet. She is fatigued and has a poor appetite. Her facial complexion is pale white as are her nails and the undersides of her eyelids. Her memory is impaired and she has trouble sleeping. When she gets fatigued, she experiences heart palpitations. Her pulse is moderate or relaxed (*i.e.*, slightly slow) and fine. Her tongue is enlarged and very pale with thin, white fur. The patient also says she bruises very easily for no apparent reason. Her pattern discrimination is:
a. Spleen qi vacuity
b. Spleen yang vacuity
c. Heart blood-spleen qi vacuity
d. Spleen-kidney yang vacuity
e. Heart yin vacuity

Answer: ___

629. The guiding formula for the above case is:
a. *Gui Pi Tang* (Restore the Spleen Decoction)
b. *Liu Jun Zi Tang* (Six Gentlemen Decoction)
c. *Si Wu Tang* (Four Materials Decoction)
d. *Shen Ling Bai Zhu San* (Ginseng, Poria & Atractylodes Powder)
e. *Tian Wang Bu Xin Dan* (Heavenly Emperor Supplement the Heart Elixir)

Answer: ___

630. If there were premature greying of the hair and intestinal dryness constipation, what two medicinals might you add to the above formula:
a. Radix Achyranthis Bidentatae (*Niu Xi*) & Fructus Lycii Chinensis (*Gou Qi Zi*)
b. Radix Polygoni Multiflori (*He Shou Wu*) & Semen Cannabis Sativae (*Huo Ma Ren*)
c. Herba Cistanchis Deserticolae (*Rou Cong Rong*) & Rhizoma Alismatis (*Ze Xie*)
d. Fructus Immaturus Citri Aurantii (*Zhi Shi*) & Rhizoma Cimicifugae (*Sheng Ma*)
e. Semen Cannabis Sativae (*Huo Ma Ren*) & Semen Pruni (*Yu Li Ren*)

Answer: ___

631. If the patient has a tendency to loose stools and no sign of bruising or bleeding, what medicinal might you remove from the above formula:
a. Radix Auklandiae Lappae (*Mu Xiang*)
b. Radix Polygalae Tenuifoliae (*Yuan Zhi*)
c. Radix Astragali Membranacei (*Huang Qi*)
d. Gelatinum Corii Asini (*E Jiao*)
e. Radix Angelicae Sinensis (*Dang Gui*)

Answer: ___

Answer Key

Exterior-resolving Medicinals

1. A	13. A	25. E	37. D
2. A	14. A	26. A	38. B
3. E	15. C	27. A	39. A
4. B	16. C	28. B	40. A
5. A	17. A	29. B	41. B
6. D	18. D	30. C	42. B
7. B	19. B	31. B	43. D
8. E	20. B	32. E	44. D
9. C	21. C	33. C	45. B
10. E	22. D	34. E	46. A
11. C	23. A	35. D	47. C
12. B	24. D	36. C	48. D

Heat-clearing Medicinals

49. B	64. A	79. D	94. B
50. C	65. A	80. C	95. D
51. A	66. E	81. B	96. A
52. A	67. B	82. D	97. A
53. C	68. B	83. C	98. C
54. A	69. C	84. E	99. B
55. B	70. B	85. B	100. A
56. C	71. A	86. A	101. D
57. C	72. C	87. B	102. D
58. E	73. A	88. E	103. B
59. A	74. C	89. B	104. C
60. B	75. B	90. C	105. B
61. A	76. D	91. E	106. A
62. C	77. E	92. E	
63. D	78. A	93. E	

Downward Precipitating Medicinals

107. C	111. A	115. D	119. B
108. B	112. D	116. B	120. E
109. B	113. B	117. B	121. A
110. A	114. A	118. C	

Damp-dispelling Medicinals

122. B	126. E	130. B	134. B
123. D	127. C	131. A	135. E
124. C	128. B	132. D	136. C
125. A	129. A	133. E	137. C

138. E	144. B	150. A	155. B
139. A	145. D	151. D	156. D
140. D	146. C	152. A	157. D
141. E	147. E	153. A	158. C
142. C	148. A	154. B	
143. A	149. D		

Wind Dampness Treating Medicinals

159. D	162. E	165. E	168. B
160. B	163. E	166. A	169. A
161. D	164. C	167. C	170. E

Phlegm-transforming, Cough-stopping Medicinals

171. C	179. A	187. D	195. B
172. D	180. C	188. A	196. C
173. A	181. E	189. D	197. C
174. C	182. B	190. C	198. D
175. A	183. D	191. B	199. B
176. B	184. A	192. C	200. B
177. C	185. B	193. C	201. D
178. A	186. C	194. A	

Food-dispersing Medicinals

202. E	204. D	206. E	208. C
203. E	205. E	207. A	

Qi-rectifying Medicinals

209. B	214. E	219. C	224. D
210. A	215. D	220. A	225. B
211. B	216. A	221. E	226. B
212. C	217. C	222. B	227. E
213. E	218. D	223. D	228. A

Blood-rectifying Medicinals

229. F	237. D	245. D	253. E
230. B	238. A	246. A	254. C
231. A	239. B	247. A	255. D
232. A	240. B	248. E	256. A
233. C	241. E	249. D	257. C
234. C	242. D	250. C	258. B
235. A	243. E	251. C	259. C
236. C	244. A	252. B	260. A

261. C	264. E	267. C	270. C
262. A.	265. E	268. C	271. B
263. C	266. C	269. A	272. C

Interior-warming Medicinals

273. E	279. C	285. E	291. B
274. B	280. C	286. B	292. B
275. B	281. C	287. A	293. E
276. E	282. D	288. D	294. C
277. E	283. B	289. C	295. A
278. D	284. B	290. B	296. B

Qi-supplementing Medicinals

297. A	302. C	307. C	312. C
298. C	303. E	308. C	313. C
299. D	304. B	309. A	314. B
300. E	305. D	310. E	
301. D	306. A	311. D	

Blood-supplementing Medicinals

315. C	320. E	324. C	328. A
316. B	321. A	325. B	329. D
317. D	322. E	326. D	330. D
318. B	323. B	327. C	331. A
319. C			

Yang-supplementing Medicinals

332. A	335. B	338. A	341. B
333. C	336. C	339. C	342. A
334. C	337. B	340. D	

Yin-supplementing Medicinals

343. C	346. B	349. B	352. E
344. B	347. C	350. A	353. C
345. E	348. D	351. C	354. C

Astringing & Securing Medicinals

355. C	358. C	361. C
356. D	359. A	362. A
357. A	360. E	363. C

Spirit-quieting Medicinals

364. D	368. E	372. D	376. D
365. A	369. D	373. B	377. C
366. C	370. A	374. D	378. A
367. E	371. D	375. A	

Wind-extinguishing, Liver-leveling Medicinals

379. B	383. B	387. C	391. D
380. B	384. B	388. E	392. B
381. C	385. B	389. C	
382. B	386. D	390. A	

Orifice-opening Medicinals

393. D	395. B	397. C	399. E
394. E	396. C	398. E	

Medicinals for External Application

400. D	402. C	404. A	406. A
401. B	403. D	405. E	

Miscellaneous Questions on Medicinals

407. D	428. C	449. E	470. A
408. E	429. A	450. A	471. E
409. A	430. B	451. E	472. A
410. B	431. E	452. E	473. C
411. C	432. C	453. B	474. A
412. D	433. D	454. D	475. D
413. B	434. E	455. C	476. B
414. A	435. A	456. B	477. A
415. A	436. B	457. A	478. B
416. B	437. B	458. A	479. B
417. C	438. D	459. A	480. D
418. C	439. C	460. C	481. D
419. B	440. B	461. B	482. A
420. A	441. E	462. A	483. B
421. E	442. C	463. D	484. C
422. B	443. A	464. B	485. B
423. B	444. A	465. A	
424. A	445. C	466. B	
425. C	446. B	467. D	
426. D	447. C	468. A	
427. A	448. B	469. C	

Formulas

486. A	499. B	512. C	525. F
487. A	500. D	513. C	526. A
488. B	501. A	514. E	527. A
489. C	502. D	515. B	528. D
490. B	503. C	516. A	529. D
491. E	504. C	517. D	530. E
492. A	505. C	518. A	531. C
493. C	506. B	519. C	532. C
494. C	507. C	520. E	533. B
495. B	508. B	521. D	534. D
496. E	509. A	522. C	535. B
497. D	510. A	523. C	536. E
498. C	511. D	524. E	537. D

Additions & Subtractions

538. A	547. A	556. B	565. A
539. A	548. B	557. C	566. A
540. C	549. D	558. D	567. D
541. C	550. C	559. E	568. E
542. D	551. E	560. A	569. C
543. B	552. A	561. B	570. E
544. E	553. A	562. B	571. C
545. D	554. C	563. D	
546. E	555. A	564. C	

Categorizing

572. C	578. B	584. A	590. A
573. E	579. D	585. C	591. B
574. A	580. C	586. B	592. C
575. B	581. E	587. D	593. E
576. B	582. B	588. E	594. C
577. E	583. B	589. B	

Treatment Principles

595. A	598. E	601. B	604. C
596. D	599. B	602. D	605. A
597. E	600. A	603. C	606. C

Case History Questions

607. A	614. A	621. C	627. E
608. D	615. C	622. A	628. C
609. D	616. C	623. B	629. A
610. C	617. F	624. E	630. B
611. D	618. D	625. F	631. D
612. E	619. B	626. D	
613. E	620. C		

Bibliography

The following bibliography is not necessarily the source of all the questions in this book. However, it does represent the major English textbooks on Chinese materia medica, formulas, and the writing of individualized prescriptions. It is provided as a guide to further research and study. If one studies the books below, they should have little trouble answering any of the questions in this book.

Materia Medica

Chinese Herbal Medicine: Materia Medica by Dan Bensky & Andrew Gamble, Eastland Press, Seattle, 1993. This is the "industry standard" when it comes to descriptions of the basic Chinese materia medica. Under each entry you will find the temperature, flavors, channel-enterings, functions, indications, combinations, dosages, and contraindications of all the most important Chinese medicinals. However, even though this book is huge, it still only presents the basic information on each medicinal considered standard in the People's Republic of China today.

Oriental Materia Medica: A Concise Guide by Hong-yen Hsu *et al.*, Oriental Healing Arts Institute, Long Beach, CA, 1986. This book is a pharmacopeia similar to Bensky & Gamble's above. The information it contains under each herb is not as complete, but it contains many more medicinals. Therefore, it is the next place to look when Bensky & Gamble do not list a particular Chinese medicinal you are trying to find out about.

A Barefoot Doctor's Manual, revised & enlarged edition, Cloudburst Press, Mayne Isle, 1977. This book is a bit dated, but it does contain a large selection of Chinese materia medica. One of its useful features is that it includes many alternative names for each medicinal. This can be useful when translating from Chinese, since Chinese authors do not always use the contemporary standard name.

The Divine Farmer's Materia Medica: A Translation of the Shen Nong Ben Cao translated by Yang Shou-zhong, Blue Poppy Press, Boulder, CO, 1998. This is the *locus classicus* of the Chinese materia medica literature and is one of the three or four foundation texts of Chinese medicine. In it, readers will find very early descriptions of Chinese medicinals written from an avowedly Taoist point of view. This book provides a useful comparison with modern, standard Chinese medicine's descriptions of the same medicinals.

Handbook of Chinese Herbs and Formulas, Vol. 1: Materia Medica by Him-che Yeung, self-published, LA, 1985. This is the first volume of a two volume set. It is another basic materia medica. Its information is less complete than Eastland Press's standard text, but is a good cross-reference for a slightly different opinion about dosages, indications, contraindications, etc.

Legendary Chinese Healing Herbs by Henry C. Lu, Sterling Publishing, Inc., NY, 1991. This book is a fun way to begin learning about Chinese herbal medicine. It is full of interesting and entertaining anecdotes about Chinese medicinal herbs.

Dui Yao: The Art of Combining Chinese Medicinals by Philippe Sionneau, Blue Poppy Press, Boulder, CO, 1997. This book discusses 100 of the most clinically reliable two and three medicinal combinations. After one has memorized the basic information about single medicinals, going on to learn these famous, essential combinations is a great intermediate step before tackling formulas. The best formulas tend to be made from the building blocks of these combinations and these combinations are also what are mainly used when modifying prescriptions. Therefore, this is a very useful book.

Pao Zhi: An Introduction to the Use of Processed Chinese Medicinals by Philippe Sionneau, Blue Poppy Press, Boulder, CO, 1997. This book discusses the differences in clinical application of the same medicinal when used in differently processed forms. In other words, by processing medicinals before they are decocted, one can help target their clinical functions and effects more precisely. Author Sionneau goes so far as to say that differently processed forms of a single medicinal are actually different ingredients.

Formulas

Chinese Herbal Medicine: Formulas & Strategies by Dan Bensky & Randall Barolet, Eastland Press, Seattle, 1990. This is the companion volume to Bensky & Gamble's materia medica. It is the industry standard for descriptions of all the main Chinese medicinal formulas. Under each entry, it gives the ingredients and their dosages, functions, indications, dosages and administration of the formula as a whole, and cautions and contraindications of all the most important Chinese formulas.

A Clinical Guide to Chinese Herbs and Formulae by Chen Song Yu & Li Fei, Churchill Livingstone, Edinburgh, 1993. This book contains basic information on Chinese medicinals as individuals, the main Chinese medicinal formulas, and the Chinese medicinal treatment of the most common diseases. Compared to the above books, this book is essentially meant as a textbook for a *course* on Chinese herbal medicine. In that case, the above books become reference texts for the *practice* of Chinese herbal medicine.

Seventy Essential TCM Formulas for Beginners by Bob Flaws, Blue Poppy Press, Boulder, CO, 1994. This book discusses the 70 key Chinese medicinal formulas which form the core curriculum at the Chinese provincial medical colleges in the PRC today. If one learns these 70 formulas and how to modify them with additions and subtractions, one can treat almost any case. These are generally considered the most important formulas in Chinese medicine today since they are the clinically most reliable.

How to Write a TCM Herbal Formula by Bob Flaws, Blue Poppy Press, Boulder, CO, 1993. This book explains the step-by-step process of moving from a pattern discrimination to treatment principles and thence to the selection of a guiding formula. After selecting this guiding formula, it then explains how to modify that prescription to fit the individual patient. This methodology is highly dependent on the correct use of technical Chinese medical terminology and hinges on treatment principles correlated with formulas' and medicinals' categorization.

Handbook of Chinese Herbs and Formulas, Vol. 2: Formulas by Him-che Yeung, self-published, LA, 1985. This is the second volume in this two volume set. It is a basic formulas and prescriptions compendium. Its information is less complete than Eastland Press's standard text, but is a good cross-reference for a slightly different opinion about functions, indications, contraindications, etc.

Practical Traditional Chinese Medicine & Pharmacology: Herbal Formulas by Geng Jun-ying *et al.*, New World Press, Beijing, 1991. This book contains many useful charts showing what symptoms are caused by what disease mechanisms and what medicinals in a formula are combined for what purpose. Its information is succinct and easily accessible.

A Compendium of TCM Patterns & Treatments by Bob Flaws & Daniel Finney, Blue Poppy Press, Boulder, CO, 1996. This book discusses Chinese herbal formulas and their modification from the point of view of pattern discrimination. In professionally standard contemporary Chinese medicine, the patient's pattern discrimination is the most important thing, while their disease is of relatively secondary importance. If one knows what formula to use for all the main patterns of disharmony, then one can treat the full range of disease no matter how long its Latin or Greek Western medical name.

Fundamentals of Chinese Medicine by Nigel Wiseman, Paradigm Publications, Brookline, MA, 1985. This is a basic textbook on Chinese medicine covering everything from introductory theory to acupuncture and Chinese medicinal treatments based on pattern discrimination. It uses the same terminology and methodology as this book and so is a good supplementary reference for study. It is our preferred basic Chinese medical textbook.

The Heart Transmission of Medicine by Liu Yi-ren, translated by Yang Shou-zhong, Blue Poppy Press, Boulder, CO, 1998. Written in the 19th century, this book is meant to be a primer on the clinical practice of Chinese herbal medicine. Intended to be memorized and not just read, it contains very concise explanations of how to use and modify the main formulas of Chinese medicine. Using this book, one can quickly build the foundation of an effective clinical repertoire of formulas to meet the needs of a wide variety of cases.

Terminology

English-Chinese Chinese-English Dictionary of Chinese Medicine by Nigel Wiseman, Hunan Science & Technology Press, Changsha, 1995. This book is not really a dictionary since it does not contain definitions. Actually, it is only a glossary. However, it is the source for the translational terminology used in this and other Blue Poppy books. Using this book, the reader can find the Chinese characters and Pinyin for any terms used in this book.

A Practical Dictionary of Chinese Medicine by Nigel Wiseman & Feng Ye, Paradigm Publications, Brookline, MA, 1998. This is the book which defines the English language terms in the glossary above. In it, students and practitioners alike will find out the clinical implications of technical terms such as counterflow, upbearing, out-thrusting, depression, glomus, and concretions. To insure that clinicians do not overlook this book, the author included Chinese medicinal formulas and treatment strategies for all the main and minor patterns of contemporary Chinese medicine and for all the traditional Chinese disease diagnoses. Therefore, this book is a goldmine for students and practitioners alike. Its authoritative scholarship should set the new standard of education in this profession.

OTHER BOOKS ON CHINESE MEDICINE
AVAILABLE FROM BLUE POPPY PRESS
3450 Penrose Place, Suite 110, Boulder, CO 80301
For ordering 1-800-487-9296 PH. 303\447-8372 FAX 303\245-8362

A NEW AMERICAN ACUPUNCTURE by Mark Seem, ISBN 0-936185-44-9

ACUPOINT POCKET REFERENCE ISBN 0-936185-93-7

ACUPUNCTURE AND MOXIBUSTION FORMULAS & TREATMENTS by Cheng Dan-an, trans. by Wu Ming, ISBN 0-936185-68-6

ACUTE ABDOMINAL SYNDROMES: Their Diagnosis & Treatment by Combined Chinese-Western Medicine by Alon Marcus, ISBN 0-936185-31-7

AGING & BLOOD STASIS: A New Approach to TCM Geriatrics by Yan De-xin, ISBN 0-936185-63-5

AIDS & ITS TREATMENT ACCORDING TO TRADITIONAL CHINESE MEDICINE by Huang Bing-shan, trans. by Fu-Di & Bob Flaws, ISBN 0-936185-28-7

BETTER BREAST HEALTH NATURALLY with CHINESE MEDICINE by Honora Lee Wolfe & Bob Flaws ISBN 0-936185-90-2

THE BOOK OF JOOK: Chinese Medicinal Porridges, An Alternative to the Typical Western Breakfast by Bob Flaws, ISBN0-936185-60-0

CHINESE MEDICAL PALMISTRY: Your Health in Your Hand by Zong Xiao-fan & Gary Liscum, ISBN 0-936185-64-3

CHINESE MEDICINAL TEAS: Simple, Proven, Folk Formulas for Common Diseases & Promoting Health by Zong Xiao-fan & Gary Liscum, ISBN 0-936185-76-7

CHINESE MEDICINAL WINES & ELIXIRS by Bob Flaws, ISBN 0-936185-58-9

CHINESE PEDIATRIC MASSAGE THERAPY: *A Parent's & Practitioner's Guide to the Prevention & Treatment of Childhood Illness* by Fan Ya-li, ISBN 0-936185-54-6

CHINESE SELF-MASSAGE THERAPY: The Easy Way to Health by Fan Ya-li ISBN 0-936185-74-0

A COMPENDIUM OF TCM PATTERNS & TREATMENTS by Bob Flaws & Daniel Finney, ISBN 0-936185-70-8

CURING ARTHRITIS NATURALLY WITH CHINESE MEDICINE by Douglas Frank & Bob Flaws ISBN 0-936185-87-2

CURING DEPRESSION NATURALLY WITH CHINESE MEDICINE by Rosa Schnyer & Bob Flaws ISBN 0-936185-94-5

CURING HAY FEVER NATURALLY WITH CHINESE MEDICINE by Bob Flaws, ISBN 0-936185-91-0

CURING HEADACHES NATURALLY WITH CHINESE MEDICINE, by Bob Flaws, ISBN 0-936185-95-3

CURING INSOMNIA NATURALLY WITH CHINESE MEDICINE by Bob Flaws ISBN 0-936185-85-6

CURING PMS NATURALLY WITH CHINESE MEDICINE by Bob Flaws ISBN 0-936185-85-6

THE DAO OF INCREASING LONGEVITY AND CONSERVING ONE'S LIFE by Anna Lin & Bob Flaws, ISBN 0-936185-24-4

THE DIVINE FARMER'S MATERIA MEDICA (*A Translation of the Shen Nong Ben Cao*) by Yang Shou-zhong ISBN 0-936185-96-1

THE DIVINELY RESPONDING CLASSIC: *A Translation of the Shen Ying Jing from Zhen Jiu Da Cheng,* trans. by Yang Shou-zhong & Liu Feng-ting ISBN 0-936185-55-4

DUI YAO: THE ART OF COMBINING CHINESE HERBAL MEDICINALS by Philippe Sionneau ISBN 0-936185-81-3

ENDOMETRIOSIS, INFERTILITY AND TRADITIONAL CHINESE MEDICINE: A Laywoman's Guide by Bob Flaws ISBN 0-936185-14-7

THE ESSENCE OF LIU FENG-WU'S GYNECOLOGY by Liu Feng-wu, translated by Yang Shou-zhong ISBN 0-936185-88-0

SHAOLIN SECRET FORMULAS for Treatment of External Injuries, by De Chan, ISBN 0-936185-08-2

STATEMENTS OF FACT IN TRADITIONAL CHINESE MEDICINE by Bob Flaws, ISBN 0-936185-52-X

STICKING TO THE POINT 1: A Rational Methodology for the Step by Step Formulation & Administration of an Acupuncture Treatment by Bob Flaws ISBN 0-936185-17-1

STICKING TO THE POINT 2: A Study of Acupuncture & Moxibustion Formulas and Strategies by Bob Flaws ISBN 0-936185-97-X

A STUDY OF DAOIST ACUPUNCTURE & MOXIBUSTION by Liu Zheng-cai, ISBN 1-891845-08-X

TEACH YOURSELF TO READ MODERN MEDICAL CHINESE by Bob Flaws, ISBN 0-936185-99-6

THE SYSTEMATIC CLASSIC OF ACUPUNCTURE & MOXIBUSTION (*Jia Yi Jing*) by Huang-fu Mi, trans. by Yang Shou-zhong & Charles Chace, ISBN 0-936185-29-5

THE TAO OF HEALTHY EATING ACCORDING TO CHINESE MEDICINE by Bob Flaws, ISBN 0-936185-92-9

THE TREATMENT OF DISEASE IN TCM, Vol I: Diseases of the Head & Face Including Mental/-Emotional Disorders by Philippe Sionneau & Lü Gang, ISBN 0-936185-69-4

THE TREATMENT OF DISEASE IN TCM, Vol. II: Diseases of the Eyes, Ears, Nose, & Throat by Sionneau & Lü, ISBN 0-936185-69-4

THE TREATMENT OF DISEASE, VOL. III: Diseases of the Mouth, Lips, Tongue, Teeth & Gums, by Sionneau & Lü, ISBN 0-936185-79-1

THE TREATMENT OF DISEASE, VOL IV: Diseases of the Neck, Shoulders, Back, & Limbs, by Philippe Sionneau & Lü Gang, ISBN 0-936185-89-9

THE TREATMENT OF DISEASE, VOL V: Diseases of the Chest & Abdomen, by Philippe Sionneau & Lü Gang, ISBN 1-891845-02-0

THE TREATMENT OF EXTERNAL DISEASES WITH ACUPUNCTURE & MOXIBUSTION by Yan Cui-lan and Zhu Yun-long, ISBN 0-936185-80-5

260 ESSENTIAL CHINESE MEDICINALS by Bob Flaws, ISBN 1-891845-03-9